AF412754

THE PATIENTS' BOOK

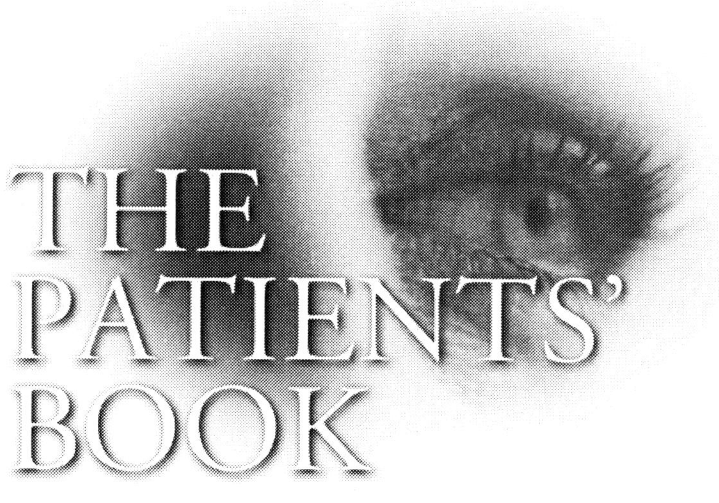

BY SANDRA MᶜCRAY
AND DIANE HARTMAN

Book and Cover Design by Michael Mahoney, Soliloquy Graphics

FIRST EDITION

ISBN: 0-9678647-3-9

How important is this book?

Two recent reports have highlighted serious problems with the U.S. medical system.

In one of the reports, the inspector general of the Department of Health and Human Services noted that the FDA has "no quality control system" to detect dangerous side effects from prescription drugs. The FDA's voluntary reporting system is not working. Few doctors, pharmacists, and hospitals, report adverse reactions to drugs.

The second report by the Institute of Medicine at the National Academy of Sciences provided evidence of the extent of medical errors. Consider the opening paragraph of the Executive Summary:

> *The knowledgeable health reporter for the Boston Globe, Betsy Lehman, died from an overdose during chemotherapy. Willie King had the wrong leg amputated. Ben Kolb was eight years old when he died during "minor" surgery due to a drug mix-up.*

And, based on data from hospitals:

> *...at least 44,000 Americans die each year as a result of medical errors. ...the number may be as high as 98,000. More people die in a given year as a result of medical errors than from motor vehicle accidents (43,458), breast cancer (42,297), or AIDS (16,516).*

The tip of the iceberg

According to the committee:

- *These figures offer only a very modest estimate of the magnitude of the problem since hospital patients represent only a small proportion of the total population at risk....*

Recommendations

Here are some of the specific recommendations of the committee:
1. Congress should create a Center for Patient Safety.
2. A nationwide mandatory reporting system should be established that provides for the collection of standardized information ... about adverse events that result in death or serious harm.
3. The development of voluntary reporting should be encouraged.
4. Health care organizations should focus greater attention on patient safety.
5. Performance standards and expectations for health professionals should focus greater attention on patient safety.
6. The FDA should increase attention to the safe use of drugs.
7. Health care organizations and the professionals affiliated with them should make improved patient safety a declared and serious aim.

Our first thoughts on reading these recommendations were: isn't patient safety already the primary objective of health care organizations, professionals, and the FDA? If not, what other goals are these organizations and professionals pursuing? And why?

How can we meet the goal of patient safety?

We believe that the goal of patient safety must begin with patients and include education and training. A federal agency can help this process by allocating money for patient education programs and by mandating the collection of data reflecting medical errors and adverse drug reactions and releasing that data in a form that patients can understand. It would be unthinkable for our government to hide the existence of airplane crashes, along with the reasons for the crash. Yet, that is what is happening now with medical errors. Once this information is released on a continuous basis, patients will become motivated to take more control over their health care.

In the final analysis we must be prepared to count on ourselves to assure that we get the best possible care. This book will show you how.

Table of Contents

About the Authors

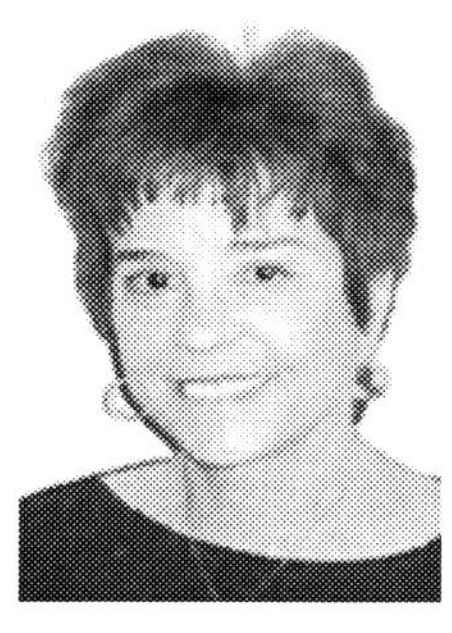

Sandra B. McCray. Sandy is a retired lawyer and the founder and executive director of Colorado HealthSite (formerely Colorado HealthNet). She works as a full time volunteer for Colorado HealthSite.

In large part, this is a book about Colorado HealthSite, an electronic health information service for people with chronic illnesses. My partner in this book, Diane, and I met on Colorado HealthSite.

Colorado HealthSite arose out of my experience getting through a serious illness. I was born with kidney disease. Although the disease caused constant urinary tract and kidney infections, sometimes requiring hospitalization, I never understood that I had any role in the management of my disease. I now believe that my passivity contributed to the loss of my one fairly good kidney, leading to a kidney transplant and two total hip replacements. It is true that my doctors failed to ask some important questions and did not listen as well as they should have. Yet, what I have learned is that once I finally decided to take control of my health, I found wonderful doctors.

In Chapter 5, I recount my story before I became an involved patient. My story today is very different. In my fifties, I started reading and researching about kidney dialysis and transplant. That my life is good now is due to several things:

- *The wonders of modern western medicine, which gave me a new kidney when my last one failed.*
- *Harsh, but effective, pharmaceutical drugs that reversed my body's initial rejection of my new kidney and still continue to suppress my body's immune system so that it won't reject the kidney again.*

- *Modern medicine that gave me two new hips when the anti-rejection drugs caused avascular necrosis, collapsing both of my hips.*
- *My personal decision to be an active partner in my health care.*

As I became a more involved patient, I began to tell my doctors that I wanted to be a partner in my care. Most responded positively. I left those that didn't. Two surgeons and one generalist stand out in my mind today. I chose the surgeons only after meeting with them and asking the questions I drafted after lots of research. Dr. Arthur Matas and the team at the University of Minnesota kidney transplant center always had time to answer my questions before and after my transplant. They taught me how to read my own blood tests to monitor the function of my new kidney. They saw me through a nasty rejection "episode." Dr. Eric Johnson at the UCLA orthopedic surgery center spent several hours with me before my hip replacements, carefully answering the questions that I had marked in my big book on hip replacement from the National Institutes of Health and did a superb job of replacing my hips. I also have a very special "gateway" doctor. Dr. Sharman Hurlow is a careful listener and excellent clinician who is not reluctant to call in a specialist when necessary.

At the time I was facing the loss of my kidneys, there was no book telling me how to research my illness, how to ask questions of my doctors, how to get a diagnosis, how to learn about my medications. There were no web sites to help me find information and support groups. Diane and I wrote this book to enable you to do these things.

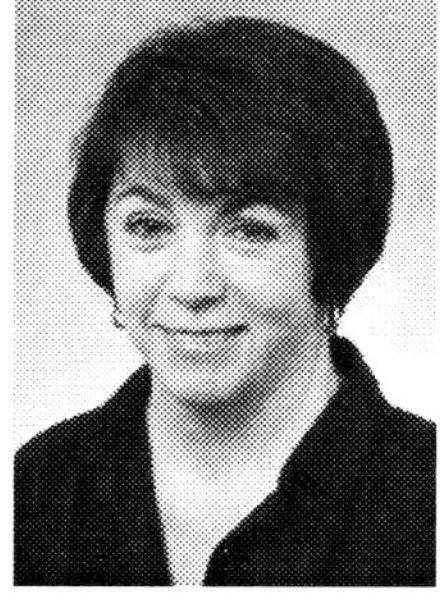

DIANE HARTMAN. Diane is a former journalist and educator and now works in public relations.

I met Sandy when I looked at Colorado HealthSite and was so impressed with what she has done. I was curious about any information she had about hip replacements. It's been hard to get information from doctors about what I can and can't do since this operation.

We became friends and soon talked about writing this book together. I wanted to be a part of it with the hope that I would learn to do what we're writing. Too often, I've been afraid to question the judgments and opinions of doctors. I've had doctors who treated me as an equal, were kind and gentle, helped me educate myself and some who actually encouraged me to talk. I've had doctors who were sarcastic, arrogant, condescending, careless and incompetent. I now know that my own preparation and my own attitude can make a huge difference in what happens to me.

I firmly believe that we're in a different era of health care and that we're not going back. Nobody cares as much about my health as I do, and if I don't take responsibility, nobody else will.

Introduction

This is not another "self-help" book, nor is it a book for all patients. It's for anyone with a chronic or acute illness who wants to consider this question: Am I willing to go all the way to come out "whole" - whatever your definition is - from my illness?

Who wouldn't?

We know a woman who took a self-defense course because she lived in a high-crime area. The first thing her instructor asked was whether she would do ANYTHING to save her own life or that of a loved one. At that point, the woman decided she would do whatever it took to save her life or that of her child. Some of the other women hesitated; they weren't so sure. It isn't always an easy decision.

We believe this life is worth fighting for and enjoying to the fullest extent, as long as we can. You have to make the determination up front and then re-commit along the way. If you wait to decide until you're midway though a bone-marrow transplant, a major organ transplant or breast cancer treatment, you may be in too much pain or be too depressed to marshal your mental and emotional defenses.

If you are willing to go all the way to come out physically, mentally, emotionally or spiritually whole from your illness, this book is for you and the support team you will build. The book will help you educate yourself in ways you may not have imagined, help you learn how to communicate with your doctors, and will describe the psychological tools you will need. We want you to gain strength from the tools offered.

We will tell you our stories, as well as the stories of other survivors, their caregivers and support team members. We will describe strategies used by other patients to develop a long-term successful relationship with their doctors. We will give you checklists to keep your thinking on track and help you organize your resources. We will ask you to make your own lists and questions. **We will, in short, ask you to be an assertive and involved patient.**

Here are five areas we will emphasize:

1. Many parts of our current medical system are inadequate. Despite its enormous power, modern medicine does not have all the answers, particularly in connection with chronic illnesses. You need to understand the shortcomings in our system and how to deal with them if you want to avoid becoming a victim of those defects. (Chapters 1 and 2)
2. Patients have to take responsibility for themselves by being honest with themselves and their doctors and following an agreed-upon treatment plan. (Chapter 3)
3. Once diagnosed, you need to learn as much about your illness and treatment as you can. (Chapter 4) Probably the quickest place to learn about your illness is on Colorado HealthSite (www.coloradohealthnet.org). (Chapter 5)
4. Begin building a support team as soon as you are diagnosed with a serious illness. You're going to need help. You're going to need one or more people to help you consider options, to give you comfort and support, to tell you when you're not being logical, someone to listen and empathize, and maybe to fix you some soup. You need to be clear with that person that he/she should be your strong representative, that she should question your medications, ask about procedures. We call this the Buddy System. (Chapters 6 and 7)

5. There are things we want doctors to know - it's our patient's agenda. Part of our agenda includes what we think should be done on a national level. (Appendix I).

A note about anger.

We know patients and caregivers who are very angry at the care they or a loved one has received. Anger is often a response to pain and helplessness; it can be a response to the unfairness of being afflicted with a life-changing illness. For many people anger is the fuel that helps them be assertive with medical personnel, allows them to take charge of their own care, and gives them a sense of control. Anger can feel like a power surge.

At some point, you might visualize anger as a positive gift and transform it into energy you can use for your health and well being. As you move along, the anger may start to get in your way. Angry people don't always make the best decisions or see the whole picture objectively. Moreover, anger is not a healing emotion. When it's of no use anymore, consider giving it up and directing your energy to the job at hand - taking care of yourself in a new phase of your life.

Read this book with a buddy.

After we had written a draft of this book, we got together with other patients who were intimately involved with chronic and acute illnesses. They read the book and discussed it with us in focus groups. They gave us feedback, good and bad. One woman surprised us by saying: "This book isn't for the faint of heart."

The more we listened to the members of our focus groups, the more we remembered our own experiences and the more we knew that we wanted to make a big point right away: If you're about to take a medical "journey," you need a "buddy."

When you first suspect something is not quite right, when you get shocking test results back, when you find a suspicious mole or a lump, or even if you just have a nagging idea that you should see a doctor, we hope you'll think about who among your friends and family could help you.

Some of us think we should be able to walk this path alone or that there's really no one to turn to. Please think again. You're going to need help. After you read this book, ask your friend or friends to read it also.

You may need someone to go to the doctor's office with you, to hear nuances of a diagnosis you may not be ready to hear, to ask questions you may be avoiding. You'll need a friend to bounce your decisions off, someone who can say: "let's look at your options," and hardest of all, someone who can help you examine your decisions. You may get depressed; a friend can spur you into taking some action that may relieve the depression. We'll be talking about support systems throughout the book.

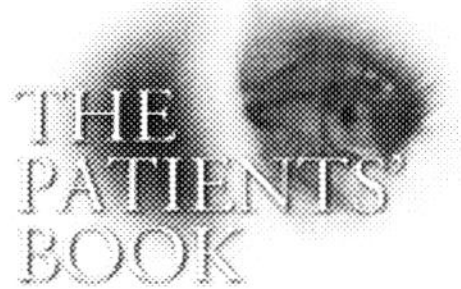

CHAPTER 1

Personal Challenges

While our goal is a physician-patient partnership, we know that both physicians and patients set up barriers that make such a partnership hard to develop. Here we describe some of the personal barriers that keep us from that goal as well as the benefits to patients who push those barriers aside.

Aggressive Doctors

The passive-aggressive model is hard to give up. We all know that it is far easier to do our jobs if we are in control. If you are a doctor, it is even harder to give up control once you have spent many years in professional training. Then, instead of putting your training to work efficiently, you must listen to questions from lay people challenging your prescribed remedy. Moreover, the managed care company you work for has only allotted 15 minutes per patient and you simply cannot do an exam and answer all these questions in that time. Now, add in yet another frustration. Assume that your remedy is correct and agreed to by your patient (stop smoking or lose weight), yet your patients continue to engage in the very behavior that is making them ill. It's enough to make you want to find another profession.

Doctors are often accused of wanting to play god with their patients, but the problem may be more than an oversized ego. The so-called god complex may be a generous instinct gone awry. One doctor told us that when he graduated from medical school, he was ready to save the world with his prescription pad. When he found out that he did not have a remedy for the world's ills, this doctor was able to make the transition into a doctor-patient partnership. Many doctors have not and some cannot.

Passive Patients

Some of us are passive by nature, so we will have to work very hard if we want to play a role in our health care. Others of us are passive only in the face of medical "expertise." We know many people (male and female) who are good at their jobs and assertive in their relationships at work and socially. Yet, when they walk into their doctor's office they simply cannot ask even one question. Their minds become blank.

While they are in the office, they start to think:

(a) their doctor is an expert,

(b) he or she has the patient's best interest at heart,

(c) the various pains they are feeling throughout their body are "not really that bad" after all,

(d) the worrisome side effects of their drugs are really not worth mentioning,

(e) their doctor is very busy and has many sick people to help, so we shouldn't take up valuable time.

We have asked ourselves and others why we lose confidence when we are in our doctors' offices. Sometimes, the answer is simple. At one time or another we have been chastised by a physician who has told us we are overreacting to small discomforts or that our illness is "psychological" and we really need a therapist.

Sandy's story:

I recall one such devastating incident, just before I lost my last kidney. I told my nephrologist that I was scared, that I didn't want to go on dialysis and face a life of being tied to a machine with at best a three-year life span. Here is how he answered me (honest!): "Oh whine, whine, whine — it is always the women and it is always late in the day." Although I couldn't speak, I did have just enough courage to walk out before the tears came.

Sometimes, our passivity is our response to our doctor's language. Many physicians use medical jargon to describe their diagnosis, prognosis, and prescription. We cannot understand what we're being told, but we are sure that the words mean something and that is enough. In this game, both doctor and patient are hiding behind medical jargon. A physician might hide behind medical jargon for many reasons, including: she is not a "good communicator" by nature and has not been trained in medical school to communicate with patients; she wants to show off her medical expertise; he is simply not aware that he is using medical jargon; he wants to dismiss the patient quickly and move on to the next one.

Some doctors combine the spoken language with body language that says "our time is short." We have heard from many patients that their doctors never enter the "exam" room, but stand in the doorway, reminding us that they are very busy, and we shouldn't take too much time.

Patients are hiding too. We are hiding the fact that we don't have the tools and courage to discuss our illness with our doctors. We may be afraid of the truth. We may know what we feel in our bodies, but we lack the vocabulary that will make us heard. When we are silent in the face of medical jargon, we aren't being chastised, but we are being ignored. And we are participants!

What's in it for us?

Given how much institutionalized and personal resistance we must overcome to claim our role as an assertive and involved patient, we'd better be sure the benefits are significant. They are!

The first benefit is that many studies show patient outcomes are far better when patients understand and are involved in their treatment.

The second benefit is that assertive and involved patients will be more alert for medical mistakes and oversights that could be life-threatening. By paying attention and taking responsibility, you can literally save your own life.

The evidence mounts:

- Adverse Drug Reactions/Hospital Mistakes.

    A recent study of U.S. hospital patients showed that adverse drug reactions kill an estimated 100,000 persons a year. An additional 1.6 to 2.6 million people face serious injury as result of adverse drug reactions. One hospital discovered that 50 percent of its adverse reactions were preventable — including 42 percent that occurred because patients were given too much medicine for their weight and kidney function. The researchers said the "best way to be protected is to be a well-educated patient and be your own advocate by asking questions and reading the information provided with prescriptions."

• Medical Errors

In late 1999, the Committee on Quality of Health Care in America at the Institute of Medicine, National Academy of Sciences, released a report describing the present state of the U.S. health care system and urging reforms. With surprising candor, the committee gave us much evidence of an alarming problem. Using hospital data, the committee estimated that:

> *...at least 44,000 Americans die each year as a result of medical errors. ...the number may be as high as 98,000. More people die in a given year as a result of medical errors than from motor vehicle accidents (43,458), breast cancer (42, 297), or AIDS (16,516).*

According to the committee, these numbers represent just the tip of the iceberg:

> *These figures offer only a very modest estimate of the magnitude of the problem since hospital patients represent only a small proportion of the total population at risk....*

The most common categories of medical errors are:

- Diagnostic – including error or delay in diagnosis, failure to employ indicated tests, use of outmoded tests or therapy, failure to act on results of monitoring or testing.

- Treatment – including error in the performance of an operation, procedure, or test; error in administering the treatment; error in the dose or method of using a drug; avoidable delay in treatment or in responding to an abnormal test; inappropriate (not indicated) care.
- Preventative – failure to provide treatment, inadequate monitoring or follow-up of treatment.

Medication errors in particular are common and are often preventable. Inappropriate prescribing is an important factor in accounting for medication errors. Here are some examples of inappropriate prescribing:

- physicians do not routinely screen for potential drug interactions, even when medication history information is readily available.
- pharmacists dispense the wrong drug or wrong strength,
- physicians prescribe inappropriate drugs for nearly a quarter of all older people,
- hospitals order and /or administer the wrong medications.

- ## Patient/Support Team Stories

Sandy's story:

"After my kidney transplant, I had pain in my left leg and thought there was something wrong. Since I have had trouble with blood clots in the past, I thought that might be the problem. I asked for an ultrasound to check it. The result came back negative, but the pain persisted. After years of dealing with doctors, however, I have learned to be pushy. I

insisted on a second ultrasound and a different technician to read it. So, I had another one the next morning. This time a different technician did the study and reported the results — a 6-inch clot!"

Diane's story:

Every day in the hospital after hip replacement surgery, someone from my surgeon's office would come by my bed, put a hand on the bottom of my foot and push toward me. "Any pain?" he would ask. "If that ever hurts, you could have a blood clot." It never hurt.

Five weeks after surgery, my leg did begin to hurt. After a few days, I had a temp of 102, more pain than I'd ever experienced, my leg looked swollen and discolored – and if you pushed my foot, it hurt. I went to the surgeon's office after taking two pain pills. As I walked on crutches down the hall, I heard several nurses say: "Yep, she's got a clot. Look how purple her leg is." But a few minutes later, three medical people (not my surgeon, but what I guessed were a physician's assistant, a nurse and perhaps a doctor) said they didn't think I had a clot. "Why do I have fever? Why does my leg hurt so bad?" I asked. One told me I probably had a cold. I told him: "I'm afraid I have a clot. I'm afraid I'll die." He replied: "Well you could and you might, but I don't think so."

I went home and remember thinking I shouldn't move around so the clot wouldn't break free (I knew nothing about clots.) A wonderful neighbor called early the next morning: I was in bed crying from the pain, feeling helpless. She suggested we go see my GP. My doctor took a look, said she believed I did have a clot, and sent me for an ultrasound, where they found the clot in my upper leg. She hospitalized me immediately.

As I checked in, the hip surgeon appeared like magic. He never apologized for his staff, there was never anything that sounded remotely like "I'm sorry we didn't listen to you."

Looking back, I wonder how I could have doubted myself, and all the evidence. Why didn't I insist on an ultrasound that afternoon? Later, I said to the hip doctor: "Are you going to take this experience back and discuss it with the staff so it won't happen again?" Oh yes, he replied.

Sara's Story:

My mother-in-law was 89 years old and suffering from chronic pain from two sources: her intestines which had been damaged from radiation treatments for ovarian cancer 25 years before, and a deteriorated hip damaged from the prednisone she had to take to control the diarrhea and intestinal pain. We were trying to take care of her at our home, but there was a crisis with unremitting pain which led us to call an ambulance and take her to the emergency room. Although they could find nothing new, they admitted her to the hospital for observation which was a relief to us because we were exhausted from trying to care for her at home.

After she was moved to her room, a nurse came to give her a shot. She explained that it would help her absorb calcium. I thought that a little odd, given what was wrong with her, but thought maybe it would help her hip. I asked the nurse to explain it again to my mother-in-law because she was hard of hearing and in so much pain that she was not able to understand very well. The nurse explained it again. By this time, I was quite suspicious and asked which patient the shot was for. The nurse looked at her card and said the name of someone else, not my mother-in-law. My mother-in-law's name was printed very clearly in large letters over her bed. I told the nurse that I thought she had the wrong patient. She at first objected. I told her my mother-in-law's name and asked her to look at the card over her bed. She checked again and realized that the shot was for the patient across the hall.

Needless to say, I was upset because we had taken her to the hospital because we were exhausted and frightened. Now, I realized I could not leave her alone at the hospital even for an hour. This underscored for me the importance of having a family member or close friend or private duty nurse or someone present in the patient's room most, if not all, the time to watch the staff and advocate for the patient who may be too old, too medicated, too weak, or not conscious and therefore unable to advocate for herself.

Disenfranchised and Disfavored Patients

We define here a class of patients who are neglected and/or under-treated. The class includes those who are uninsured, underinsured, poor, or elderly.

You may wonder how we can urge you to become an assertive and involved patient if you lack access to the health care system or if, having access, you are consistently mistreated by that system? And what are the benefits to you of becoming involved?

The numbers of people who suffer from health system defects is daunting, so we focus on two such patients who will serve as representatives of this class.

Lynnette is a disenfranchised patient. She is a 32-year-old woman with severe Lupus. She is African-American, a group that is at special risk for Lupus. For many years, Lynnette had no insurance.

Lynnette's story:

I became an uninsured person a year ago when my employer went through reorganization, eliminating several positions and taking away some of my responsibilities. I was offered extended health insurance but because I had not yet found another job, I could not afford the increased insurance premiums. I began working for a temporary agency and benefits were not offered until you had worked consistently for at least nine months and the coverage wasn't good. After about six months of temporary positions, I finally landed a job on my own. Unfortunately, after about six weeks I experienced a Lupus flare that was attacking my liver and I became so ill that I could not work. I was hospitalized and because my employer could not keep my position open for what turned out to be a lengthy recovery, I resigned. I had not completed the 90-day probationary period, so I had no health insurance.

When you don't have insurance or the right kind of insurance, many options are not open to you. Doctors neglect to inform you what medications or procedure will help if you're not covered. I have needed operations to re-cement my hip replacements for about a year. My knees lack blood flow so they have to be replaced as well. I have been told that if the situation is not rectified soon, there might not be enough bone to work with. But without insurance, no doctor is willing to work with me, preferring to use the Band-Aid approach and put me in a wheel chair until I acquire some.

My doctors insist that their hesitation to do something has nothing to do with my lack of insurance but if my situation is so dire, why the hesitation? I have been approved for disability payments but have had no insurance for two years. I don't qualify for SSI, which would provide me with medical insurance because my husband earns too much.

I pay cash for all of my medications, which average about $250 a month. I see my doctors only if I think the situation is something I can't handle. If I don't feel well, I self medicate by increasing my steroids, take antibiotics and daily doses of calcium, acidophilus and vitamins. I keep a diary of what I eat and try to keep my appetite up because I have a tendency to lose my appetite when I am on a low dose of steroids. I buy nothing for myself because my medications cost so much. I also research my condition to see what I can do for myself versus going to a doctor. My husband and children assist me with all of the household duties and I have become a prisoner in my home because I cannot go out on my own. I have very little contact with the people I used to socialize with because my disabled status makes them uncomfortable.

Later, we will tell you more about Lynnette and what she is doing on the Internet to help herself and others. Her story is truly inspiring.

Our second disenfranchised/disfavored patient is Carrie, an elderly patient. It may surprise you that we have included the elderly in the disenfranchised and disfavored class of patients. Aren't most elderly patients covered by Medicare? Maybe so, but our discussions with elderly patients have uncovered serious problems in their health care, even when they are able to afford what Medicare excludes. So, we call this group "disfavored."

Consider the following list of drugs prescribed for and taken by Carrie, a relatively healthy 87-year-old woman who walks two miles a day and does yoga three times a week:

- Lanoxin,
- Premarin,
- Provera,
- Tambacor,
- Lipitor, and
- Fosamax

Although Carrie is just 5'1" and weighs less than 115 lbs., none of the dosages are tailored to her size and age. The dosages prescribed for her are identical to those that would be prescribed for a 40 or 50-year-old male or female weighing much more. Many of the drugs she takes have special instructions, such as take only with food, take only one hour before or two hours after a meal, take only at night, take only with a full glass of water, etc. A 40-year-old would have a hard time managing this drug regime. Asking a 87-year-old to do so would be laughable if it weren't so commonplace.

Should Carrie have been prescribed these drugs? It is true that her total cholesterol is high, but her HDL cholesterol is also very high (a good sign) and her triglycerides are normal. Her complete lipid profile does not place her at high risk (see Colorado Health-Site for more about this issue and how you can calculate your own risk). It is also true that she has moderate osteoporosis, but recent studies have shown that Fosamax has very serious side effects for the women taking it, particularly those over the age of 75. Even more important, there are several other drugs with bone-building properties that have fewer and less serious side effects.

Is it possible for the disenfranchised and disfavored to take advantage of the advice in this book?

Yes. For example, Lynnette and Carrie represent several of these categories. They had an uphill battle, but each has made progress in becoming a more assertive and involved patient.

Lynnette uses the Internet to research her illness and has become an advocate who interacts with other patients on the Colorado HealthSite Lupus Forum for patients. She writes and publishes book reviews on health related issues. Carrie is not comfortable with the Internet, but she reads medical health news letters, discusses the issues with others, and has become a health awareness advocate in her retirement community.

We have structured this book to include Lynnette and Carrie and others like them, as well as those who fall within the traditional community of patients.

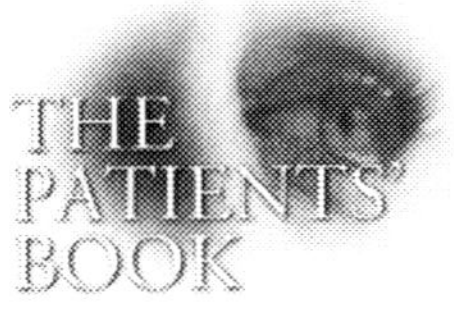

Chapter 2

Modern Medicine: Three Barriers to a Doctor-Patient Relationship

What patients want most from their doctors is simple to state:

- Listen to us
- Believe us
- Work with us
- Go the distance with us

In many cases this isn't happening. Who is to blame? Many deserve a share of the blame:

- doctors who think that they are the keepers of all medical knowledge and wisdom,
- patients who won't take responsibility to educate themselves and change their harmful behavior,
- insurers who limit the amount of time that patients and doctors can spend together, and
- an embedded medical system designed only to treat diseases, not patients.

In this chapter, we focus on the "system" component of the problem.

Many people forget that the current system was not always in place. There was a time when doctors used to come to a patient's home (you may not remember that!). In that setting, family members, friends, and local healers all felt they could offer an opinion about what was causing the sickness. Back then, treatments were designed for a particular patient, not for a class of diseases. In his essay, "Body and Mind in Nineteenth-Century Medicine," Charles Rosenberg noted that 19th century doctors practiced a form of holistic medicine, focusing on knowing their patients and their environments, including their home and families.

This changed when all the special tools and machines used to diagnose and treat were in one place — and the patient had to travel to them. In the new era, the role of the physician changed dramatically and with it the physician-patient relationship.

Consider the following quote from a renowned doctor - Dr. Jacobi - who was part of the "new" era:

"What the patient has to tell you constitutes precisely the least important part of what you must learn about him in order to be able to understand his case, and to do him any good," because only the physician can "understand the pathological significance of one symptom as compared to that of another."

When all the scientific machines and doctors were gathered in one place, we began to trust them instead of ourselves. They had the knowledge and the studies; we didn't. They used big words; we struggled to understand. They doled out potions; we took them.

We wouldn't want to go back to early medicine, but we would like to see the doctor-patient relationship more balanced.

In our view, there are three components of the current system that work to keep the balance askew:

1. the over reliance on "standard treatment protocols,"
2. the emphasis on double-blind, placebo-controlled studies that lead to a dismissal of important anecdotal patient evidence, and
3. the use of drugs as primary therapy to cure all ills.

These three components save time because doctors are not required to individualize treatments. We are well aware that standard treatment protocols, double-blind/placebo controlled studies, and pharmaceutical drugs have played a key role in advances in medical treatments. But, as in many disciplines, success often has a darker side - in this case, the loss of the patient's story, making it hard, if not impossible, to develop a physician-patient partnership.

At the end of this chapter, we describe some alternative medical treatments that foster a stronger physician-patient relationship.

1. The Problem with Standard Treatment Protocols

Doctors have standard procedures for certain illnesses (called "protocols"). If you have X disease, you get the standard medicine or treatment for X — a long way from the days when doctors treated patients as individuals.

If you are diagnosed with one or more of the common chronic illnesses, you'll probably be handed a printed booklet or "action plan." (You may, instead, not get a diagnosis at all, but we deal with that subject in the next chapter).

There is ample evidence that most patients who receive a diagnosis and treatment plan from their doctors don't or can't follow them without training and on-going support. A look at one chronic illness — asthma — illustrates some of the problems.

A person with asthma has to understand his or her illness and manage it. Asthma is chronic and won't go away. Over the years, the National Institutes of Health has published several standard treatment protocols for asthma. These protocols are very helpful to doctors because they are developed by well-proven statistical techniques with large populations of asthmatics. They tell doctors when the asthma patient should see a specialist, the levels of severity and kinds of drugs that should be prescribed at each level, and what patients need to know to manage this condition.

The standard protocols are less helpful for patients because, while they represent a baseline level of care, they are overly simplistic and don't take into account the kinds of help that asthmatics need to manage their illness. So, we are not surprised that the protocols have failed us. Despite these protocols, the number of asthma cases and the mortality from asthma has increased sharply in the last decade, particularly among children. The death rate for children 19 years and younger increased by 78% between 1980 and 1993. In 1990, costs related to asthma were estimated to total $6.2 billion; the projected cost of asthma in the U.S. for the year 2000 is expected to double to $14.5 billion.

Recent studies also show that both doctors and patients are not complying with the protocols.

What's going on here?

- 83% of doctors say that they prescribe peak-flow meters (a device that allows patients with chronic asthma to monitor their condition) but only 28% of asthma patients actually have one, and only 9% report using one at least once a week;

- 70% of doctors say they prepare a written action plan for all, most, or some of their patients, but only 27% of patients say that they've ever seen a written action plan.

What about our national asthma treatment goals?

A recently completed (1998) large survey of asthma sufferers and doctors showed that asthma care in America falls far short of national treatment standards. Fewer than one in ten patients could name asthma's underlying cause; and half of the patients surveyed believed that they could treat only asthma attacks, not their underlying cause as recommended.

One obvious problem here is a large communications gap between doctors and patients. We believe that excessive reliance on standard treatment protocols increases this communications gap.

Physicians, already under pressure to treat patients quickly, may feel that they have done their job by handing their patients a written action plan.

Patients, unable to understand or unwilling to comply with the action plan, may not tell their physicians that they are not following the plan. What patients need is help with motivation, help in finding support groups and buddy plans, and follow-up care.

There is another problem with reliance on standard treatment protocols. Again, we will use asthma as an example. Some studies place blame for the growth in the number and severity of asthma cases on the increase in external and indoor allergens, such as environmental pollutants, animal dander, and cockroaches. Indoor allergens are controllable in large part. But a physician who doesn't know his or her patient and who is physically removed from the patient's home and work environment may not know what is going on at home. It is interesting to think about the effect that physician home visits might have on the discovery of indoor allergens.

The Centers for Disease Control agrees that standard treatment protocols for asthma are not enough. Their asthma agenda includes the following:

- Promote healthy home environments
- Translate science into public health practice
- Provide patient and community-level education and develop prevention partnerships.

These goals begin to get at the problem - the need for patient-oriented and personalized medicine. We believe that the CDC agenda should be incorporated into the standard treatment protocols, starting with at least one home visit for each asthma patient.

2. The emphasis on tightly controlled research studies and the failure to listen to and learn from patient stories

We understand the scientific method and the importance of objective evidence to support the use of a treatment or drug. We are glad that prescription drugs go through rigorous testing (double-blind, placebo controlled studies) before they are given to us. In fact, we believe that in some cases today, drugs are approved too quickly for use in the general population.

Yet, the disdain with which we hear some doctors talk about the uselessness of anecdotal evidence (patient stories) disturbs us. The failure to listen to patient experience with a particular treatment or drug can have serious consequences.

Sandy's story:

In 1994, I began taking cyclosporin, prednisone, and azathioprine to keep my body from rejecting my transplanted kidney. After 4 years, my blood tests showed that my liver function was beginning to be impaired. My doctors believed that the cause was the azathioprine and so told me to switch to CellCept. I had read lots of information about CellCept and knew that it had some added benefits, including possible protection against chronic rejection. So, I was happy to accept the change. After about a week, however, I woke up with my eyes crusted over and painful. The diagnosis? Conjunctivitis. During the next 2 months I had 3 more cases of conjunctivitis, an eye inflammation that I hadn't had since I was very young.

Although none of my doctors agreed with me that CellCept was the problem and although the published description of the side effects of CellCept did not include conjunctivitis and dry eyes, I believed that CellCept was the culprit. So, I stopped CellCept and went back to azathioprine. The conjunctivitis stopped but the liver tests continued to show problems. Then, newer evidence showed that CellCept may be beneficial for long term retention of transplanted kidneys. Finally, I went to a new ophthalmologist, who treated lots of transplant patients. I told him my story and my guess as to the cause. He confirmed that he had talked to many transplant patients who had continual conjunctivitis who said that CellCept seemed to be one of the problems. He told me that the conjunctivitis that these transplant patients had was not infectious conjunctivitis but keratoconjunctivitis sicca or dry eyes conjunctivitis. The very fact that he could give me a diagnosis boosted my confidence in him. He also offered me a quick solution that he said worked with many transplant patients. He could plug some or all of my tear ducts, either partially or fully, so that the lubricating tears would not drain out, leaving me with dry eyes. Since the procedure was a 5-minute office procedure and completely reversible, I had two tear ducts partially plugged. I am back on CellCept, this time with fewer problems.

I am grateful to this superb clinician who listened to and learned from his patients, rather than relying solely on the double-blind/placebo controlled studies. Perhaps someday the collective experience of transplant patients with CellCept and dry eyes will be tested in a rigorous study. Until then, however, we patients need this information so that we can take this valuable drug without the harmful side effects.

This isn't, of course, just a story about the nuisance of conjunctivitis. It is a story about saving Sandy's kidney by finding a way for her to take a drug that would not harm her liver and would give her the best chance to avoid chronic rejection. Sandy was lucky enough to finally find a doctor who understood her problem with CellCept, but relying on chance is risky. This ophthalmologist worked with lots of transplant patients. He knew about the problem, his partners knew, and their patients knew. But, no other doctor that Sandy asked knew.

In our view, one of the major reasons for the failure of our current system to handle chronic illnesses is the isolation in which our clinical doctors work. Medical journals are reluctant to publish anecdotal evidence learned from patient stories. So, much of what clinicians and patients need to know has not been systematically gathered and distributed. In its reliance solely on academic research, modern medicine has lost sight of the value of anecdotal experience, to the detriment of both clinicians and patients.

3. The Overuse of the Prescription Pad

In this section, we focus on prescription drugs. We believe, however, that the same issues exist with the use of herbs and dietary supplements and our recommendations are the same in both cases.

Many physicians are quick to pull out their prescription pad to cure their patients. Other therapies like behavior modification require individualized treatment plans and take more time than drug therapy.

The result? Doctors and patients have come to believe that there is (or will soon be) a miracle drug for all of our illnesses and discomforts. We know clinically obese patients who believe that they don't have to worry about their weight because there will soon be a drug that will either:

(a) allow them to lose weight painlessly while eating all they want, and/or

(b) cure or control the illnesses that are commonly correlated with obesity - diabetes, heart disease, or cancer - despite their weight.

Recently, drug companies have begun using the media to push new "miracle" drugs to the public. Have you noticed the recent upsurge of TV ads for prescription drugs? The ads picture beautiful, healthy-looking people interacting in gorgeous scenery. Often the ads use a well-known athlete, newscaster, or entertainer to sell the product. The side effects are mentioned in passing in a lilting voice that assures us that they occur in only a small fraction of those who take the drug. These ads have been enormously successful for the drug companies. Despite the fact that sometimes there is no mention of the illness that the drug will fix, hundreds of thousands of us have rushed to our doctors to get a prescription. What you may not have noticed is the increase in FDA warnings about serious side effects of many of the new drugs. These warnings are not seen by most patients. We will tell you how to find the warnings in Chapter 5.

Will our doctors give us the prescription we ask for? Listen to Lynnette, our young friend with Lupus:

"Doctors are so quick to treat you with a pill. My medicine cabinet is a virtual pharmacy. It's a good thing I don't have an addictive personality because my doctors will pretty much give me anything."

We call this reliance on drugs the "magic bullet" conspiracy. The co-conspirators include:

- doctors, who on their own or with pressure and money from pharmaceutical companies, increasingly offer drugs to the chronically ill without first trying a more benign approach,
- drug companies that push their wares on TV, in magazine ads, and increasingly pay doctors large fees to enroll patients in trials,
- HMOs and insurance companies that don't pay for patient education and motivation and even actively promote certain drugs through deals with drug companies,
- the FDA, which condones drug company advertising directed at the public;
- the National Institutes of Health, which funds many drug research studies but few behavior modification studies; and
- patients.

Yes, patients are willing participants in the conspiracy. We have accepted, even welcomed, the idea that all of our ailments can be fixed with a drug, herb, or vitamin. Any other view might require us to question our physicians and alternative healers, live with some physical discomfort, and become active participants in our healing, such as losing weight, exercising, participating in stress reduction, and eating right.

Our reliance on drugs and herbs has lots of drawbacks. None of these remedies is without side effects, either alone or as a result of interactions. There are now so many drugs and so little research about the long-term effects of the drugs and their interactions with other drugs, herbs, and supplements that we are literally risking our lives when we ask for and/or accept our doctor's prescription without question. If we are, as we believe, a nation of over-medicated consumers, then what is the alternative? After all, most of us don't take prescription drugs for recreation. We take them because we have an illness that requires some medication or because we are in pain.

Is there a better way?

The answer ranges from yes to maybe. So little money is spent on behavioral modification research that we can't give a complete answer to the question about a better way. Recently, however, two articles appeared in the Journal of the American Medical Association that described the results of two studies that compared treatments consisting of behavioral modification with drug therapy. A third study in the same journal demonstrated how the simple act of writing about the stressful experiences in illness resulted in significant reduction of symptoms in patients with asthma and rheumatoid arthritis. Here are our summaries of these three studies:

Study 1. Treatment of urinary incontinence in older women

In this study, the behavioral modification therapy was an unqualified success — well accepted, easy to follow, and with no side effects.

To get a quick sense of the enormous problem of urinary incontinence in the U.S., listen to these facts and statistics:

- More than 15 million people in the U.S. have urinary incontinence,
- Urinary incontinence is more prevalent than diabetes,
- Approximately 38% of women older than 60 suffer from urinary incontinence,
- Incontinence predisposes patients to other health problems, contributes to depression and social isolation, is a significant source of dependency among the elderly, and is widely cited as a factor in nursing home admissions.

The study group consisted of 197 women aged 55 - 92 years. The subjects were randomly placed in one of three treatment groups: one group was given a placebo, a second group was given drug treatment, and the third group participated in biofeedback-assisted behavioral treatment.

Nearly 97% of patients in the behavior modification group reported being comfortable enough with the behavioral intervention to continue it indefinitely. Moreover, these patients did not suffer any of the adverse effects common with pharmacological intervention. In contrast, over 75% of those who received drugs said they wished to receive another form of treatment.

Despite the success of the behavioral therapy, the medical community continues to treat urinary incontinence with drug therapy and drug companies continue to advertise their urinary incontinence drugs on TV. What are the reasons for the use of drug therapy when safer and less expensive alternatives exist? Drugs use less physician time; individualized treatments take more.

What should be the role of the doctor here? We know that doctors are not trained in patient motivation and behavior modification techniques in medical school. We think that, at least in connection with chronic illnesses, medical schools might do well to add those disciplines to their curriculum. Until that happens, we believe that doctors should tell their patients about these options and steer them to professionals who are trained in these behavior modification techniques.

Study 2. Intensive lifestyle changes for reversal of coronary heart disease

In this study, the behavior modification therapy was a qualified success — the lifestyle changes required were very demanding, but the outcome for those who did comply was very positive.

Forty-eight patients with moderate to severe coronary heart disease were placed in one of two groups: a control group and an experimental group. The required lifestyle changes made by the participants in the experimental group included:

- a 10% fat vegetarian diet,
- moderate aerobic exercise,
- stress management training,
- smoking cessation,
- group psychosocial support.

The results of the study were dramatic - there were more than twice as many cardiac events per patient in the group that didn't change their lifestyle than in the group that did follow the lifestyle changes. Also, the life-style change group had a marked reduction in the frequency, severity, and duration of angina after one year, which was sustained at five years. This study showed that patients who undergo comprehensive lifestyle changes can dramatically cut their risk of coronary atherosclerosis without the use of drugs, angioplasty, and other common therapeutic procedures.

Listen carefully to what these two studies tell us. We are given and are taking drugs despite the fact that behavioral modification therapies are often safer, less costly, and more effective. We are given drugs because writing a prescription is easier and requires less physician time, and we are given drugs because we lack the self-discipline to change our lifestyles.

Study 3. Effects of Writing About Stressful Experiences on Symptom Reduction in Patients With Asthma or Rheumatoid Arthritis

This study demonstrated the beneficial effects of the simple act of writing about stressful experiences. One hundred seven volunteer participants completed the study. Each of the participants had either asthma or rheumatoid arthritis as confirmed by physician diagnoses. The participants were divided into two groups. Members of the experimental group were assigned to write about the most stressful event of their lives. Members of the control group were told to write about emotionally neutral topics. Typically, the latter group's writing assignment involved a time management topic to reduce stress. All participants were asked to write for 20 minutes on 3 consecutive days a week. The writing took place in private rooms to ensure confidentiality. The disease activity outcomes were evaluated at the beginning, at 2 weeks, 2 months, and 4 months. Here are the results:

• Approximately 47% of the experimental patients improved,

- Approximately 24% of the control group improved.

Here is how the editorial described the importance of the study: "Were the authors to have provided similar outcome evidence about a new drug, it likely would be in widespread use within a short time. Why? We would think we understood the 'mechanism' (whether we did or not) and there would be an industry to promote its use. Manufacturers of paper and pencils are not likely to push journaling as a treatment addition for the management of asthma and rheumatoid arthritis. But the authors have provided evidence that medical treatment is more effective when standard pharmacological intervention is combined with the management of emotional distress. In short, 'it is clear that mind matters'."

The Importance of Patient Power in Chronic Illnesses

In our view, managing a chronic illness requires:
- disciplined and motivated patients,
- physicians who help educate their patients,
- support staff to monitor compliance and motivate patients.

We also believe it's necessary to:
- place curbs on drug advertising to the public, and
- spend more research dollars on behavioral therapies to determine what works and what doesn't.

Today, many physicians do not view education and support as part of their job. They place blame for noncompliance on the patient, who is said to lack motivation. We believe that noncompliance is a failure of both parties — the physician and the patient. The physician has failed to educate and support his or her patient, and the patient has failed to accept personal responsibility for his or her part in the treatment plan.

Many doctors do not view education and support as part of their job.

Well over 90 million people in the U.S. have one or more chronic illnesses, and this number is rising rapidly as we age. The cost of chronic illness is staggering:

- chronic diseases account for at least 70% of all deaths in the United States.
- the medical care for people with chronic illnesses accounts for more than 60% of the nation's medical-care costs.

According to a recent article in the Journal of the American Medical Association, our health care system is largely based on the diagnosis and treatment of acute conditions, while the needs of those of us with chronic conditions go unmet.

There it is, pure and simple! As patients with chronic illnesses, we cannot wait passively for doctors or drugs to come to our aid. **We must meet our own needs by becoming educated and actively involved in our health care, and we must demand the tools we need to do this.**

The point is that patients with chronic illnesses want time with their doctors, and they want personalized treatment. If they don't get it from their traditional doctors, they will, if they can, find it from alternative providers, some reliable and some charlatans.

The authors are patients who owe their lives and health to traditional medical doctors, and we do not want to see the current system continue to lose credibility with patients. This book is our effort to make the system a place where patients will feel welcome enough to remain.

In the next chapter, we focus on the patient's role in making our system work better. We believe that the same rules for patients apply, whether we see alternative providers or traditional doctors, or choose to use complementary therapies or traditional medicine. In both cases, we must take more responsibility for our health. That is the topic of our next chapter.

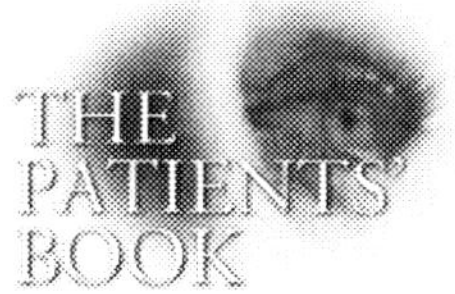

Chapter 3

Taking Responsibility for Our Health

The plans outlined in this chapter aren't for those who are acutely ill. Obviously if you're bleeding, bent and broken, in great pain, with high fever or otherwise in need of medical care, go get it.

These suggestions are for those whose symptoms creep up or don't seem to make sense.

We assume you already have a family doctor. Perhaps you didn't have a choice of doctors but must go where your managed care plan sends you. If you do have a choice, talk to your most trusted friends and family to get recommendations and then check them out - CAREFULLY!

A story from Dolores:

Our insurance plan gave us a list of doctors we could use. I didn't know any of them. I asked around at our office and one woman recommended a doctor: "He listens and he's just wonderful," she said. I went to him for several years and he was very personable. Once I asked about some rough spots on my face. "Oh, those are just pimples," he said. (A year later, I found out they were skin cancer.) When I started having hor-

rible pain in my knees and hips, he prodded my buttocks and said "Well, you're too young for arthritis and it would hurt back here if you had it." He sent me down the hall to another doctor who said I should see a bike specialist because obviously I was riding my bike wrong. It took another year to get arthritis diagnosed.

You can check credentials in several ways. For instance, get on the Internet and:

- Go to the "doctor finder": at www.ama-assn.org
- Find out about board certified medical specialists at www.certifieddoctor.org
- Ralph Nader has a site at http://www.citizen.org (they charge a fee)
- Call your State Board of Medical Examiners.

If possible, interview the doctor before you commit to what could become a long-term relationship. These questions would be appropriate:

- What's your policy on phone calls?
- How long will I get to see you when I have an appointment?
- Who stands in for you during weekends, vacation times, etc.?
- How do you feel about "complementary" therapies?
- If you think you know what's wrong, ask specific questions about your illness and treatment.
- How many diabetics or asthmatics or transplant patients (fill in your particular illness) do you treat?

Afterwards, evaluate the conversations. Did you understand each doctor? Did he/she answer your questions clearly? Were you happy with the policies?

If you already have a doctor, have been given a diagnosis and your doctor is talking to you about treatment, here are some simple questions to ask yourself when you leave an appointment. These questions are from an article in the Journal of the American Medical Association (JAMA; vol. 282; Dec. 22/29, 1999). The authors listed seven elements that should be part of the conversation a doctor and patient have so that together they can make an informed decision. How does your doctor score? Answer the questions below with yes or no.

Did your doctor discuss your role in decision making?	❏ Yes	❏ No
Did he or she discuss the nature of the decision?	❏ Yes	❏ No
Did he or she discuss alternatives?	❏ Yes	❏ No
Did he or she discuss the pros (benefits) and cons (risks) of the alternatives?	❏ Yes	❏ No
Did he or she discuss uncertainties associated with the decision?	❏ Yes	❏ No
Did he or she make sure you understood the decision being made?	❏ Yes	❏ No
Did he or she ask you about your treatment preferences?	❏ Yes	❏ No

A perfect score is seven yes answers. However, the authors of the JAMA article found that only nine percent of doctors they studied would get a perfect or high score. Remember that you have a crucial role too. If your doctor doesn't initiate these discussions, you should.

Once you're satisfied you have a good general practitioner, we think you should spend some time PREPARING for your visit to discuss the current problem you're having, so that you'll be ready to ask the right questions.

Step One: Take an inventory

If you, like most Americans, rush around a lot, you may be feeling some pain and throwing some over-the-counter medicine at it. You may also be taking herbs mixed with prescribed medications. Maybe you read in a magazine about St. John's Wort - that sounded good - so you take one of those a day.

Who knows the witch's brew you're concocting every day inside your body?

We're going to suggest that you listen to your body, but you probably already knew that.

One way to do that is to deliberately stop taking all that stuff. **(WE ARE NOT TALKING ABOUT PRESCRIPTION MEDICINE AND VITAMINS THAT YOU NEED. WE REFER TO OVER THE COUNTER SELF-PRESCRIBED HERBS AND SUPPLEMENTS.)**

Gina's story:

I was incredibly constipated, to the point that I thought I had a bowel blockage. My GP sent me to a specialist who scheduled me for a colonoscopy as an outpatient in the hospital. He did the test; when I woke up from the anesthetic, he was gone. He didn't return my phone calls for ten days. Finally, when I talked with him and asked what was wrong and what I was supposed to do, he said: "Well, you talked while I was doing the test. I told you there was nothing wrong, don't you remember?" No, I didn't remember anything - surely, from seeing many patients he knew the effect of those drugs. He did prescribe an herbal laxative, which worked okay. But months later, at my yearly checkup with my GP, she said "Stop taking all that stuff you're taking." Immediately, I stopped having any problem with constipation. I thought back and wondered why the "specialist" didn't ask me what mix of supplements, vitamins, etc. I was taking before doing an invasive test. Later, I added back some vitamins and was able to isolate the pill causing the problem.

Unless the pills, herbs, supplements, etc. you take are life saving, try giving them up for a week. Drink a lot of water and try to clear your system. And here's a big step - especially for those who are in pain - stop popping the Tylenol or Advil for a week so you can really know what's going on. You need to know how much pain you have and where it is.

Step Two: Write it down

Keep a journal for at least a week. Each day, write down exactly what's going on in your body. That may mean sitting for a few moments in the morning or evening without the TV on, not talking to the dog or a friend, not continuing to rush.

Some of the questions you might ask yourself:

- Is the pain/nausea/burning/itching constant or does it come and go?
- If not constant, what times of the day do I feel the symptoms?
- Where, specifically, is the particular symptom located?
- What seems to make the symptoms more or less intense?
- On a scale of 1 - 10, what is the intensity of the particular symptom?

- Have I had feedback from others - for instance, that I'm limping or grimacing?
- How are my sleep patterns? Eating patterns?
- Have I gained or lost weight recently?
- Do I feel isolated, depressed, over-excited, irritable?
- Do I get short of breath quickly?
- Have I been experiencing unexplained numbness?

The list need not be extensive, but you will probably be surprised that the terms you use to describe what's going on with you may match exactly the words others use — and this will help the doctor immensely.

Emma's story:

After an emergency triple bypass and a long recovery, Emma looked back and realized she had had symptoms of heart disease for years. *I had episodes of cold sweats with a lot of pain during the night; that happened more times than I want to think about. They would go away and then I didn't want to think about them anymore. I even had the "crushing pain" people talk about, but it wasn't exactly in my chest so I didn't think it could be my heart. I was in full denial. In the couple of years before the heart attack, I quit going on hikes with my family because I couldn't breathe well and it embarrassed me. I never said anything to the doctor about it.*

The "cold sweats" and the "crushing pain" are terms heart patients are familiar with. A doctor could have been tipped off by these words. Shortness of breath is also a major symptom of heart disease in women, but few people know that.

If you have some general health books (some good ones are offered to clients by HMOs and the American Medical Association puts out a very easy to read one), you could spend some time taking your symptoms and trying to match them. Don't spend too much time on this step because you do want to keep an open mind.

This brings up another suggestion for adults who want to be responsible for their health. Keep a record of your health.

- Try to remember back to childhood illnesses and write those down.

- Think about accidents, trips to the emergency room, allergic reactions to over-the-counter or prescribed medicines. As an adult, have you had operations or been diagnosed with an illness?

- What shots or immunizations have you had? What were the results of mammograms, pap smears, hearing and eye tests, blood tests? What's your cholesterol level and has it changed much? (You should know your LDL and HDL levels and the difference between them.) What's your triglyceride level, blood pressure? What drugs (legal and illegal) have you taken? Did they help you, upset your stomach, make you dizzy, work well? If female, did you take birth control pills? When did you start and how long did you continue?

- Women should try to remember (or ask siblings or parents) when they started menstruation. They should also keep records of their periods - put a star on the calendar the day you start to keep track.

- Think back and write down illnesses that your parents, grandparents had and what your grandparents and/or your parents or siblings died from.

Step Three: Check your attitude

Here are two groups of people - see if you recognize yourself.

One group, upon feeling not so good, becomes convinced a brain tumor is growing or multiple sclerosis has settled in. The other group, feeling pain, denies and rejects it and becomes even more physical, trying to work it out somehow (these are the people who say, "I'm healthy as a horse. I never get sick, etc."). We have found ourselves in each one of these groups at different times in dealing with our illnesses. Both attitudes are pretty unrealistic and can interfere with getting to the problem. Try to back away from either of these extremes.

Our advice: Take an inventory of your attitude. If your mental set is that doctors know all and they will "fix you," you're not alone. That's where most people are because we've been programmed that way. Perhaps you feel entirely different from our scenario, but it's important to know exactly what your attitude is. Knowing your own attitude puts you on the road to becoming an educated, thoughtful consumer in the health system. It's your body and your life.

It's not easy when you're in pain. But this is where you recommit: "I'm willing to go all the way to come out whole from this illness." Now you're ready to go to the doctor and do your best to help him/her get a correct diagnosis for your problem.

Step Four: Make a list

This is the piece of paper that some doctors hate to see. But your list won't be random questions; it will be based on your own experience. Begin by describing your symptoms, then ask your questions. Be courteous but persistent. Do not leave the office without answers to your questions.

The first few moments you talk to the doctor are the most important. Doctors are known to interrupt. One study has shown that during the first 90 seconds of the medical visits studied, doctors interrupted patients 69 percent of the time — after 15 seconds on average.

Another study showed that doctors ask 90% of the questions. Certainly you want your doctor to ask questions, but you also need to be asking them. This makes you involved in your own process; besides getting valuable information, patients who ask questions feel more in control, feel they have more options and have more courage.

Another phenomenon that patients sometimes engage in is "late disclosure." That's when you go through an exam, take up the allotted 15 minutes and as you walk out the door you say, "Oh, by the way doctor, I've had this pain...." This is where your list will be invaluable - you'll know what to talk about first.

This sounds simplistic, but be sure to TELL THE TRUTH. Most medical symptoms are not something we want to discuss in public. They're messy or disgusting or have to do with bodily functions we usually don't talk about. But the doctor's office is no time for shyness or hesitation - you have to do your part to help them get a diagnosis. (If saying certain things makes you uncomfortable, practice saying them before you get there.)

If we could listen in on daily conversations with doctors, you might be surprised at how many start like this:

Doctor: "How are you?"
Patient: "I'm fine."

You're not fine or you wouldn't be there! Affirm to yourself that sickness doesn't equal weakness. You don't need to put on a brave front for a doctor - in fact, it's counterproductive. This is not the time for a stiff upper lip. It's the time to say: "I hurt, right here." Very few of us want to see ourselves as unhealthy or as having done something foolish (taking drugs, drinking too much, having risky sexual relations, etc.) that could affect our health. The doctor has seen it all before - give him/her every chance to diagnose you.

After you've told the doctor what your symptoms are, based on the journal you've kept, ask for a possible diagnosis. Ask if tests are needed to rule out certain illnesses. If you are a person with a chronic illness and laboratory tests are needed, ask what the tests measure and ask your doctor to leave orders stating that you can have the results given to you by phone or FAX as soon as they are in.

Sandy gets her blood checked regularly to measure how her transplanted kidney is functioning. Her doctor has told the lab to FAX the results to her. This is VERY IMPORTANT. For those of us with chronic illnesses, part of taking responsibility for our health is to understand what our lab tests measure and what our specific lab results are. We can't become motivated to take better care of ourselves unless we understand how we are doing.

Think of it this way - to lose weight, you need a plan to eat fewer calories and exercise more and a goal. Equally important, you must know what you weigh now and what you weigh as you implement your plan to see if it is helping you reach your goal. We know that many doctors are reluctant to give patients their lab tests, so you will have to be strong. Remember, they are your tests!

If the doctor prescribes something:

- Ask whether the dose is appropriate for your age, weight, and kidney function.

- Ask about side effects and how the new drug might interact with any medications you're now taking.
- Ask how long the drug should take to work.
- How long should you take it?
- Should you take it with food or not? You might even say to your doctor: "I'd rather not take any medicine if you think I'll get well just as quickly without it." Many people go to a doctor's office, wanting to walk out with "something," and saying this might reassure the doctor you don't want to be patted on the head medicinally.
- Ask if there is any kind of special diet or special exercises you could be doing to help your condition. Are there things you should or shouldn't be doing?

A good thing to do at this point is to restate what you think the doctor has said and repeat the instructions for care. Once you start taking the drug or drugs prescribed, be sure to pay close attention to any effects you feel and to report them to your doctor.

Harriet's story:

After being diagnosed with severe osteoporosis, I was given Fosamax, which caused lots of gastro problems for me. My doctor then switched me to Didronel, which I take cyclically - 14 days on and 88 days off. I noticed that I would get depressed at about day 7 and the depression would last until the end of the 'on' cycle. The depression lifted when I was on the 'off' part of the cycle. I asked my doctor whether Didronel caused depression. He said that none of the literature mentions depression as a side effect, but that many of his patients had noticed the same thing. Although I decided that 7 days of mild depression was something I could handle, I really appreciated my doctor listening to me and telling me that he had heard the same thing from other patients. This small incident gave me a great deal of confidence in my doctor - a listener!

Step Six: Hit The "Books"

If you're lucky, your doctor has given you a diagnosis. He could be right or wrong. He could know a lot about it or not. She could know a good specialist to send you to — or not. She may have a certain philosophy when faced with this condition: treat it aggressively - or not.

David's story:

David is a young Hispanic male who has a family history of diabetes, including a mother who has lost a leg to diabetes. Because of his family history, David had a diagnostic test for diabetes. The results showed he was in the early stages of diabetes.

During his office visit, David's doctor gave him the results of the test in numbers but didn't explain what the numbers meant. Later that week, David received a booklet in the mail telling him how to manage his diabetes. When he called the doctor fearful that he had diabetes, he was assured that he didn't have diabetes. As it turned out, there were several mistakes made in connection with David's diagnosis. David's fasting blood sugar numbers were 123, which is a category that is now considered "impaired." The impaired category numbers range from 110 to 125, so David's numbers put him at the high end of this category. (A diagnosis of diabetes is made for those with fasting plasma glucose level of 126.)

The federal government is currently funding prevention studies to see if early interventions with high risk patients like David can delay or even prevent the onset of Type 2 diabetes. David's doctor didn't give him any of this information. The result was that David wasn't started on a prevention plan.

We don't mean to sound negative about doctors - they have saved our lives. They are bombarded with stacks of research material, in their particular area, every day. They can't possibly keep up on everything in their field and take care of emergencies and their regular practices. We believe this has to be a team effort, and you have to be on the team.

We believe, at this point, you need to try and learn as much as you can about what's wrong with you and the treatments for it. As you begin to research, keep these six goals in mind:

1. What is usually done to treat this condition?
2. Are there brand-new ways of treating it and are there controversies within the medical community about treatments?
3. Where are the top doctors and centers for this illness?
4. Are there associations you can turn to? (Diabetes, etc.)
5. Are there complementary therapies?
6. Where can you turn for emotional support?

One of the big points of this book is that we as patients have to take responsibility for ourselves. Even when we're in pain, facing life-threatening illnesses, or waiting for the next test — we want to have the kind of spirit within ourselves that allows us to ask questions, reject thoughtless or careless treatment, demand the truth and reach out for help when we need it.

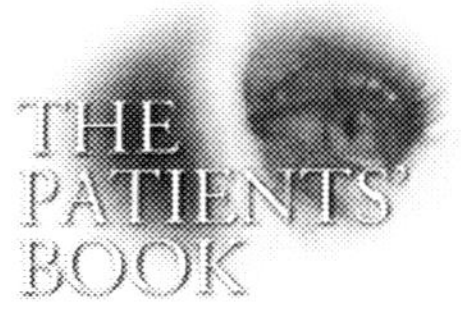

Chapter 4

Educating Ourselves: Turning to Mother Web

"For the first time, patients have a tool at their fingertips that will provide them with an enormous amount of medical information. The available and free information on the World Wide Web ranges from factual descriptions of illnesses and drugs to academic studies and clinical trials to forums where patients can learn from each other. The trick is to learn how to distinguish the good, patient-oriented sites from those sites with questionable information or that still dispense knowledge under the old model – as a form of prescription."

Sandra McCray,
Founder and Director of Colorado HealthSite.

A warning:

You will hear some warn you about bad information or outright health fraud on the Web. In fact, the "anti-web" health groups are, at this very moment, gathering forces to rid us of the "bad medicine and quack healing therapies" on the web. Do some health websites have bad information? Do some of the healer websites have a crass commercial purpose? Of course! Now, how many of you have ever had a physician give you bad information? No information? How many have ever had your doctor fail to tell you exactly why he or she has chosen a particular treatment plan or drug? How many have ever had a physician or health care provider prescribe drugs without mentioning their often serious side effects or interactions with other drugs? Enough said!

Beware of sites that masquerade as information sites.

You need to learn how to distinguish good information from bad without regard to whether the source is a MD, another patient, an alternative healer, or the Internet. We begin this section with a checklist for "bias free" and accurate information. We do not pretend that our checklist will enable you to spot all potentially biased or inaccurate information. We also realize that our checklist may lead you to label as potentially biased some information that is accurate and helpful. This is a checklist only. Its function is to raise your antennae. You will note that the checklist below tells you to watch out for sites that masquerade as information sites when they are really selling products and services. If you are looking for specific products on the web, then these sites may well be the place to go. If you are looking instead for information about a particular illness, then such sites may not be the best place to start.

Website checklist alert

Answer each of questions below "yes" or "no." A "no" answer means that the site you have found does not meet our criteria for a bias-free health information web site.

Is It Bias Free?

1. Does the website clearly state the source of the information it presents?

    ☐ Yes   ☐ No

2. Is the information on the site current (updated within the last 6 months)? Health information sites come and go on the web at a rapid rate. Many so-called "ghost" sites remain with out-dated information, even after the original creator has moved on to something else.

    ☐ Yes   ☐ No

3. If the website sells herbal remedies and dietary supplements, does it give specific warnings about drug interactions and side effects?

    ☐ Yes   ☐ No

4. If the website sells herbal remedies and dietary supplements, does it provide information explaining when certain herbs and supplements should not be used at all? One example: the negative effect of immune-boosting herbs and supplements on autoimmune diseases.

❏ Yes   ❏ No

5. Are the herbs or supplements being sold tested for purity and strength?

❏ Yes   ❏ No

This is a very serious issue. A recent study published in the New England Journal of Medicine found:

CONTAMINANTS IN DIETARY SUPPLEMENTS. *The dietary supplements contained a raw material imported from Germany and labeled as plantain. The plantain was contaminated by Digitalis Lanata, which can cause glycoside poisoning with symptoms of nausea, vomiting, and abdominal pain.*

ADULTERANTS IN SOME ASIAN PATENT MEDICINES, *including undeclared ingredients such as ephedrine and phenacetin. Lab tests done by the California Department of Health Services also revealed lead, arsenic, and mercury above the amounts permitted in oral pharmaceuticals. In fact, of the 260 products tested, 32 percent contained undeclared pharmaceuticals or heavy metals. (New England Journal of Medicine, September 17, 1998.)*

6. If the website is run by a hospital, does the hospital give you a list of the number of surgical procedures it performs annually in each specialty? Does it give you statistics on patient outcomes?

❑ Yes   ❑ No

7. If the website is run by a physician or other health care provider who is offering his or her services did he/she list his credentials and his or her success rates for the services offered?

❑ Yes   ❑ No

Finding the Information: What Search Engines Can and Cannot do

An Internet search engine is one way to find the health information you seek. To use a search engine for health information, you must pull up the search engine using its address or "URL." We give you the URLs of some of the most used search engines below. Then type the name and correct spelling of a particular illness, health institution, medication, etc. into the box provided. You can type in a phrase too. For example, if you want to know whether the drug prednisone is used to treat Lupus, you might type in "prednisone and Lupus." What a search engine does with that word or phrase is "surf" the web to find sites that have information on words or phrases that you have typed.

There are many search engines, each with their own strengths and weaknesses. Below is a list of search engines that you may find helpful. The best way to find your favorite is to do a search on a topic in each of the engines below and compare the results. To a certain extent, the choice of a search engine is personal, and a comparison test is best. As a test, type "asthma" in each of the following search engines in the list below, then scroll down through the listings that the search engine returns, and finally click on a couple of the individual sites.

- Yahoo   www.yahoo.com
- Northern Light   www.northernlight.com
- Alta Vista   www.altavista.net
- Excite   www.excite.com
- Snap.com   www.snap.com
- Google   www.google.com

Now, you can see some of the problems with search engines. Most of the problems are obvious. For example:

- Note the number of web sites that your search found for you to look at - from many thousand to several hundred thousand. Of course, you won't look at all of these sites because that would require several weeks.

- What about the search engines that give you their guides to the "best sites?" Sometimes the site owner has paid for the "best site" designation for the high visibility placement. Many of the "most visited sites" are engaged in selling goods and services, not in providing information. We have no opinion on the value of these products and services, but the sites do not meet our criteria for bias-free health information. We are never told how the search engine has determined that the sites listed are the "most visited" or "best."

- Search engines return many duplicate sites.

- Note when the site was last updated. In some cases, several years have elapsed. For some illnesses, this failure to update the site may not cause a problem; but for most illnesses a two-year or even one-year lapse renders the site useless. You will have to check even outdated sites, however, because sometimes the problem is with the search engine. More and more frequently search engines themselves have failed to update their information.

- If you click on the sites listed, you will find that many no longer exist. Health information sites on the web come and go at a rapid rate.
- Some search engines ask you to refine your search. So, for example, you can type in "asthma medications." We did that and still got hundreds of sites.

Alternatives to Search Engines

Here are some simple tips for finding up-to-date and credible information.

Government, Foundations, University Medical Center, and Medical Journal sites.

- One of the best health information sites on the web is the one developed and maintained by the National Institutes of Health. You can find their home page by typing in: http://www.nih.gov/health/. From the home page, you can click on health information and find an extensive list of specific health information to access. We give our government high marks for the job it has done so far in getting important health information out to the public.
- Some national health-oriented foundations have web sites with useful information on specific illnesses. The best of them offer free access to information and to nationwide support groups.

- Sometimes, a university medical center will have helpful information, but often the information is for public relations only. A notable exception, and in our opinion the best all around cancer site on the web, is OncoLink from the University of Pennsylvania: http://cancer.med.upenn.edu/.
- Sites with information about clinical trials can be very important for those with serious illnesses who have exhausted the treatment options offered. Many of the clinical trials sites also have a phone number or email address you can use to inquire about the trials. We urge you to call even if you don't have the means to fly out of state. You may get important information just by talking to the investigator. The largest of the clinical trials sites is Centerwatch at: http://www.centerwatch.com/studies/listing.htm. Periodically checking and calling clinical trial sites is a great task for one or more of your buddies.

Comprehensive Commercial Sites

Today there are several comprehensive commercial health information sites with lots of information. Some are well organized and easy to use. Others, however, engage in what we call "information overload." Everything is thrown into the pot. Sometimes the same information is presented in two or three different locations and sometimes the information is speculative (i.e., a study shows that a certain drug may prove helpful in controlling a particular illness). You should try these sites out and see which ones best fit your needs.

Be careful, however. Some of the commercial sites are primarily engaged in advertising products and services and have a requirement that you become a member in order to get access to the real "meat." You will be asked to give your name and email address before you access the information. Sometimes you will be asked to give the name of your illness, followed by an extensive list of questions about your illness. We don't know what the owners of the site do with this information and neither do you. If you are not comfortable with giving away your name, email address, and other information, don't sign in.

Personal Web Pages

We have found personal web pages that are very helpful. Patients who have been through a serious illness have lots to tell us about the experience that we can't learn from the "dry" facts found on institutional sites. The problem, of course, is how to find the good ones.

Sites with Forums, Chat Rooms, Questions and Answers

We have mixed feelings about sites with patient discussion groups. Patient forums and chat rooms often have good information and are a place to identify and meet the more knowledgeable and active patients, an important goal. Just as often, however, these pages become stale, repetitive, and even destructive. On one such site, a dialysis discussion group, Sandy found the patients frequently bad-tempered and their discussions full of anger and incorrect information. Even small outbursts of anger can be devastating when you are emotionally and physically fragile because of your struggle with a chronic illness. You must have the patience to find the jewels, and you must be prepared to leave a group that does not have kindness as one of its major goals.

We strongly support sites that have a Question and Answer section in which patients can query physicians. The answers are then posted on the site for everyone to see and learn from. We believe that it is important that the participating physicians are volunteers.

You have probably noticed by now that, although we have given you tips to narrow your search for health information, it is still a daunting task. In our view, what patients need is a site that gives us a complete picture of whatever illness they are researching. At the very least, a good comprehensive site should have: facts and statistics, medications and their side effects, treatments, information about related illnesses, a list of local support groups, a list of reliable links and helpful books, and a place to ask questions and read answers. Using a search engine, you can build a comprehensive site yourself by putting together all of the bits and pieces. Few of us have the time or patience to do so.

Now, let us introduce you to Colorado HealthSite.

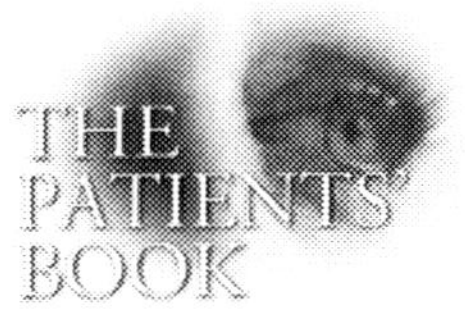

CHAPTER 5

Colorado HealthSite:
The Patients' Web Site
(www.coloradohealthnet.org)

This section is dedicated to the volunteer physicians, pharmacists, and other health care providers who answer questions and write articles for the users of Colorado HealthSite. Their generosity with their time renews our faith in our medical system.

Sandy's story

When I was facing the loss of my last kidney, there were no web sites to help me find information and support groups. Instead, I made countless phone calls to find the location of transplant statistics, then I pored through several volumes of books to determine where the best transplant centers were. I called also to locate support groups near my home. I flew to New Orleans and Florida to attend meetings of the American Association of Kidney Patients to learn about the latest in dialysis treatments and to Maryland to learn about low protein diets. I traveled to Minnesota to have my transplant and to UCLA to have my hips replaced. I was able to do all of this because my husband and I had enough money to pay my way.

Many people do not have the time or money to do the kind of travelling and research that I did. Today, however, I would be able to do nearly all of the tasks necessary to manage my illness at home by accessing Colorado HealthSite. For far less time and virtually no expense, even patients struggling with the restrictions of managed care can become educated enough about their illness to fight for good care.

Colorado HealthSite (CHS) is an award-winning health information site that was designed and developed by Sandy (see www.coloradohealthnet.org). CHS is the only comprehensive patient-oriented site on the web. It is updated daily.

As of January 2000, CHS covered 22 chronic illnesses, including:

- Arthritis,
- Asthma,
- Cancer,
- Chronic pain,
- COPD,
- Dental/Oral Health
- Depression,
- Diabetes,
- Eye Health
- Fibromyalgia,
- Heart disease,
- HIV/AIDS,
- Kidney disease,
- Lupus,
- MCS,
- Multiple Sclerosis,
- Obesity,
- Organ Transplant,
- Osteoporosis,
- Pediatric Urology,
- Sleep Disorders, and
- Stroke.

Each of the chronic illness "centers" has basic information about the illness and its management. All of the information presented is from credible sources.

Volunteer physicians answer patient questions in most of the categories covered. All of the CHS volunteer physicians are board-certified. CHS also has a drug information center with a volunteer pharmacologist to answer questions for patients. The CHS drug information center offers information about drugs and their side effects and interactions in easy-to-read format. A large holistic therapy section has extensive information about complementary therapies and a volunteer physician to answer patient questions.

Interactive sections include patient-hosted general Forums where patients can share coping skills, "Pen Pals" where patients can find email buddies with similar interests, an "Ask CHS" section for patients to ask their own questions, as well as read previous questions and answers, Patient Stories, Interviews with physicians and patients, and Book Reviews by patients of their favorite books.

Those are the basics of a very good, comprehensive website. Colorado HealthSite goes beyond the basics, however. Here are some of the "extras" that make Colorado HealthSite an exceptional and patient-friendly website;

- Each of the chronic illness information centers has a library containing the best web sites that deal with the particular illness. The library sites are chosen after extensive searches using one of the listed search engines. CHS staff updates the searches frequently and adds the best of the numerous institutional and personal web sites.

- Each of the chronic illness information centers has a "new developments" section that includes CHS abstracts of new studies and therapies from the leading medical journals. The abstracts are written in lay person's language, making them accessible to all patients.

- Each of the chronic illness information centers has a "Support Services and Resources" section that allows patients to find existing foundations and institutions that offer support for people who suffer from the particular illness covered.

- Each of the chronic illness centers has a "Related Sites" section that provides cross links patients to other illnesses that may arise as a result of their primary illness. The cross-links help patients understand the potential course of their illness and treatment and seek preventative interventions. Other cross-links take patients to the Holistic Therapies center where they can read the pros and cons of complementary therapies.

Sandy's story illustrates the importance of the cross-links:

I was born with the kidney disease of reflux. My right kidney never functioned and was removed when I was 21. My reflux remained undiagnosed and repeated infections gradually scarred my left kidney until it was gone at age 56. The long years of very low kidney function took a toll on my bones, even though I was very active all of my life. No one told me that my bones were at risk because of my kidney disease, and I never had any symptoms until after my kidney transplant and treatment for rejection. The treatment for rejection included large doses of a steroid, a known killer of bones. Then, quite suddenly (so I thought), both of my hips collapsed and had to be replaced. As I look back now, I know I should have been on a bone-building drug for decades. That is why you will find that the illnesses that may be treated with steroids – kidney disease, lupus, asthma, arthritis, organ transplant, and multiple sclerosis – are cross-linked to the osteoporosis center. Then, in the osteoporosis center, you will find a long list of CHS abstracts of studies of bone-building drugs, as well as new information on alternatives to hip replacements. Other cross-links function similarly. For example, the diabetes center has cross-links to the CHS Dental Health, Heart Disease, Kidney Disease, Obesity, Organ Transplant, and Drug Information Centers.

- An Alerts section offers patients news about problems with certain prescription drugs, as well as information about new drug therapies and treatments.
- CHS has easy to use calculators that help patients understand the meaning of their cholesterol numbers and of their body-mass index.
- CHS has a music therapy section that allows patients to become familiar with the healing power of certain kinds of music. We have found music to be an integral part of our own healing programs.
- Periodically, CHS interviews its volunteer physicians who give patients the latest information on their specialty. CHS also interviews patients who have one of the illnesses it covers. The interviews are available on line in both audio and written format.
- CHS has excellent navigational tools, including a "How to Use CHS" section and an extensive Search Engine. In the "How to Use CHS" section, users are given a written "walk-through" of the entire CHS site. This section also links patients to sites outside CHS that will help them manage their illness. For example, a link to the CHS general health information library points to medical dictionaries, clinical trials, a place to find out whether their doctor is board certified, a list of the "best" hospitals and HMOs, centers for patient advocacy, FDA warnings on herbal products, FDA consumer information, a list of the typical tests/procedures for various illnesses, Medicare information, medical alerts, health statistics and more.
- CHS's Search Engine allows users to type in a word or phrase to find where an issue is covered on CHS. CHS also has a direct link to other search engines.

- CHS works directly with patients — who "host" our general forums, write book reviews, write their own stories and stories about others who have inspired them, take our surveys, and suggest new links. We also work with doctors who answer questions, write original articles, and participate in interviews.
- CHS's librarian responds to patient users, either telling them that their question will be sent to a physician or suggesting useful sites.

Follow us now through two examples that will show the breadth and depth of information available to you on CHS.

In our first example, we begin with a person who has just received a diagnosis of asthma or whose child has just been diagnosed with asthma. We will not need to spend our time going through hundreds or thousands of sites on a search engine since we will find all that we need on Colorado HealthSite.

- What is asthma? How is it diagnosed? What are common triggers? Who gets it? How many people have it? The link on the main Asthma Center page to "Definitions, Facts, Statistics" will answer these initial questions in brief and in depth. Then, read or listen to the interviews "All About Asthma" with Dr. Jack Routes, an asthma clinician and researcher and "The Growing Epidemic of Childhood Asthma" by Dr. Andrew Liu, a juvenile asthma clinician and researcher. An interview with Clela and Aron, a mother and her asthmatic son, provides lots of practical management tips.
- Now that you have a basic understanding of asthma, you can move on to understanding how to manage your illness. The asthma management link will provide this information.

- Next, to learn about the medications commonly used for asthma patients (both adult and children), use the "Asthma Medications" link. Here you will find general information on asthma medications, as well as questions from other asthma patients and answers by CHS volunteer physicians and pharmacologists. Don't forget to read the patient and drug alerts.
- To find the best care, patients need to keep up with new developments — research into causes, as well as new treatments and medications. You will find this information in the "Asthma New Developments" link. This is a particularly important section of CHS because many doctors are not able to keep up with the latest treatments and medications. In this section, for example, you will find a large research section that includes findings on new drugs and treatments.
- Many chronically ill people feel that no one really understands what they are going through. Support groups are very helpful to overcome this feeling of isolation. Patients can find a link to support groups and resources by clicking on "Asthma Support Services and Resources."
- The "Asthma Library" offers links to the sites that the CHS staff believes are the best on the web. This one library represents well over 30 hours of web surfing and is updated frequently.
- The last two links on the Asthma main page take the user to patient questions and answers. Here, asthma patients and their friends and families can look at questions already answered and even ask their own question.

The CHS Asthma Center is designed to give patients a complete picture of asthma. It also saves the users hundreds of hours of web surfing. Colorado HealthSite uses the template described above for each of the chronic illnesses it covers. So, those of you with arthritis, diabetes, fibromyalgia, heart disease, etc., can go through the same steps to educate yourself and take control of your health.

Our second example follows the course of Sandy's illness — chronic kidney disease that led to End Stage Renal Disease (ESRD) and finally a kidney transplant. Of course, CHS did not exist when Sandy's disease developed. So, what you will read below is Sandy's recreation of her entire disease process.

Sandy's Roadmap to Becoming an Educated Patient

1. Understand the History of Your Illness.

You may wonder why it is important to understand the history of your illness. As we go along, I will point out where that understanding might have helped to change my result.

I was born with vesicoureteral reflux, probably present even before birth. So, today my first questions would be: What is reflux, how many people have it, what damage might it do? The information on the CHS Pediatric Urology Center, written by Joseph Y. Dwoskin, MD, gives a clear and complete description. Here are some excerpts:

> **WHAT IS REFLUX?** *If your child has been diagnosed with reflux, this means that during bladder filling and during voiding (urinating), some of the urine is backing up toward the kidney. Reflux is not a normal condition, and is, therefore, of concern.*

How Many Children are Born with Reflux? *The incidence of reflux in the general population is low, varying from 1 in 50 to 1 in 100 depending on the study. However, in the children with urinary tract infection (UTI), 35–50% may have reflux. The female to male ration of UTI is 3.5 to 1.*

How does Reflux Damage Kidneys? *Reflux is significant in two ways. First, if reflux is present before birth it may affect the developing kidney, as the pressure exerted by the urine can interfere with growth and development. The extent of renal damage depends on the severity of the reflux and on the time it has been present. The ureter may also be damaged by reflux. Second, infections often develop in the urinary tract that doesn't empty completely. If infected urine reaches the kidney, it can and often does cause renal infection and damage, some quite extensive.*

Unfortunately, my disease of reflux was undiagnosed. There were a couple of warning signals, but they didn't lead to a diagnosis. Recurrent urinary tract infections resulted in damage to and scarring of my kidneys. My right kidney was surgically removed when I was 21. The surgeon told my mother and me that it was small and scarred and probably had never functioned properly. Today, I know that those findings probably indicate reflux.

2. Get a medical diagnosis.

You probably already know that it can be very difficult to get a doctor to give you a medical diagnosis. We know patients who have literally begged for a diagnosis and have been told that their symptoms are all in their head and that they should consider seeing a psychiatrist. We know other patients whose doctors refuse to order tests to rule out or rule in certain illnesses like lupus, diabetes, or kidney disease.

Here is how my attempts to get a diagnosis were answered. After the removal of my right kidney, I had one remaining damaged kidney. Nevertheless, there were several points at which my left kidney might have been saved had either my doctors or I understood the problem. During my 20s and 30s I experienced repeated bladder and kidney infections. Some doctors dismissed the problem as "honeymooner cystitis" and told me that it would disappear as time went on (presumably as my body adjusted to intercourse). Frequently, when I complained of intense burning pain on urination, my doctors could not find any bacteria in my urine sample and so dismissed my complaints. The absence of bacteria in the presence of symptoms is familiar to patients with cystitis. My complaints were legitimate and signaled a serious problem that was not addressed by my doctors.

Here is the helpful information I found on Colorado HealthNet:

> (from CHS Kidney Disease Library – Interstitial Cystitis Association site, "The Ten Most Frequently Asked Questions About IC.")
>
> *#2. ... The perplexing problem is that IC patients almost consistently have at least one or more symptoms of infection, regardless of whether or not infection can be detected by conventional laboratory tests."*

With urinary tract infections that signal interstitial cystitis long term antibiotics are often necessary.

> (from CHS Kidney Disease Library – Interstitial Cystitis Association site, "The Ten Most Frequently Asked Questions About IC.")
>
> *#2. ... certainly bacterial invasions in the urinary tract will be accompanied by greater adherence and penetration of the bacteria to the underlying bladder wall. This in turn causes more severe symptoms, longer duration of the infection, and necessitates prolonged use of antibiotics which penetrate tissue rather than acting as mere antiseptics. ...*

How would I go about getting a proper diagnosis today by researching my health problems on CHS and the web?

First,

I would have told my doctors about my history and the likelihood of reflux. The reflux could then have been treated, possibly salvaging my left kidney after the right one was removed. Of course, my doctors should have asked about the condition of my right kidney. In this book, however, we focus on what patients can do to help themselves even when doctors don't do their job.

Second,

I would not accept a psycho-social diagnosis like "honeymooner cystitis." Not only is honeymooner cystitis not a disease, but the dismissal of my problems in this way made it impossible to diagnose what was really wrong and how to fix it before irreversible kidney damage occurred. Had I had the benefit of information in the CHS Kidney Disease Center Library, I could have shown my doctors that there is a relationship between sex and cystitis, but it is anatomical not psychosocial:

(from CHS Kidney Disease Library – Interstitial Cystitis Association site, "The Ten Most Frequently Asked Questions About IC.")

Answer #7: The bladder is located directly in front of the vagina, and there are many nerves between the bladder and vagina, so intercourse puts pressure on the bladder and its nerves.... Because the bladder is so close to the sexual anatomy, it's no wonder that people with bladder problems, especially Interstitial Cystitis, also have problems with sex. Many IC patients report flare-ups or symptoms during and after sexual activity.

Third,

I would tell my doctors about interstitial cystitis and insist on treatment.

- Who Gets Interstitial Cystitis?

(from CHS Kidney Disease, Library – Interstitial Cystitis Association site, "What's New.")

A recent study found the prevalence of interstitial cystitis to be more than 50 percent higher than previously reported in the U.S.. The study, conducted by Gary C. Curhan, MD, ScD, and a team of researchers from Brigham and Women's Hospital and Harvard Medical School, Boston, was designed to estimate the prevalence of IC among adult women in the U.S.. In round numbers, this raises the commonly used figure of 450,000 Americans with IC to just under 700,000.

Fourth,

I would tell my doctors that urinary tract infections often don't show up in urine cultures and that doesn't mean they don't exist.

> (from CHS Kidney Disease, Library – Diabetes and Digestive and Kidney Diseases of the National Institutes of Health, Urologic Diseases)
>
> *…Urine cultures… can detect and identify the most common organisms in the urine that may be causing symptoms. There are, however, organisms such as the bacteria chlamydia that can't be detected with these tests, so a negative culture does not rule out all types of infection…If urine is sterile for weeks or months while symptoms persist, a doctor may consider a diagnosis of IC.*

These steps might have prevented or delayed the loss of my remaining kidney.

3. Prolong the final outcome (patient activism)

Without a proper diagnosis and proper treatment, my remaining kidney continued to be assaulted by repeated infections, and I finally developed irreversible kidney disease, also referred to as End Stage Renal Disease (ESRD). None of my doctors could answer my questions as to how to get the most time out of my remaining kidney.

Nevertheless, I had a relatively normal and healthy life from my diagnosis at age 38 to the loss of my last kidney at 58. Warned at age 53 that I had at most 5 years left, I sought to prolong the life of my last kidney.

Although I was not very active in or educated about my care when I was young, by my 50s I had become knowledgeable about kidney disease and actively involved in the management of my illness.

When you are trying to find the latest news on how to slow or reverse your serious illness, the phone can be as valuable a tool as the Internet. One day, while watching TV while exercising on a treadmill, I saw a special report on the benefits of a low protein diet for patients with kidney disease. The TV commentator noted that there were trials going on at Johns Hopkins in Maryland. I called the TV station and asked for the name of the doctor who was in charge of the trials and then called Johns Hopkins and asked for that doctor. I set up an appointment and was on the plane in less than a week to discuss joining the clinical trial.

4. Make informed treatment decisions.

For several years I followed the prescribed low-protein diet. I also prepared for the inevitable — a new set of options:
- Kidney dialysis
- Kidney transplant
- No treatment

Several support groups, as well as reading about the options, helped me make my decision. The two support groups I found the most helpful are now online on CHS. In the "Kidney Disease and Dialysis, Support Services and Resources" section of CHS, you will find the American Association of Kidney Patients (AAKP) website and the website of the National Kidney Foundation.

For two years my husband and I went to the Annual Meetings of AAKP. There I met dialysis patients and transplant patients and spent hours talking with them about their choices. The meetings also provided lots of information about how to get the best life possible on dialysis, in my opinion a treatment from hell. Participation in the local chapter of the National Kidney Foundation also allowed me to meet others who had already made their choices and to learn more about the options.

Here is how the options stacked up from my viewpoint:

> (from CHS Kidney Disease Center, New Developments, "Effect of Age and Diagnosis on Survival of Older Patients Beginning Chronic Dialysis.")

Had it been available, this study would have told me that given my age at the time, dialysis came in last. I could learn here that not only is the quality of life on dialysis poor, but the average life expectancy for someone at 58 is three years. Being hooked to a dialysis machine (hemodialysis) or suffering repeated infections (peritoneal dialysis) that many endure only to buy three marginal years didn't seem to be a happy choice.

I decided that a kidney transplant ranked first, but my blood type put me low on the list, with a probable wait of three years, the life I might buy on dialysis.

5. Research important issues in medical journals.

> (from CHS Kidney Disease, New Developments, Research Studies)

At this site, I could have learned about preparing for dialysis while waiting for a transplant. There are several types of kidney dialysis, and I researched each before opting for hemodialysis. Next I researched the different kinds of vascular access. Without going into too much detail on a subject of interest only to those of us with kidney disease, I can report briefly on what I learned from reading medical journals. The best vascular access for dialysis is the "fistula," which lasts longer and has fewer infections and other complications. Yet, many doctors in the U.S. do not like to use fistulas as the vascular access since they are very hard to place. In Europe, where the survival statistics are far superior to those in the U.S., doctors use fistulas as the primary mode of dialysis access. I decided to find a surgeon who would do a fistula.

6. Accept gifts of kindness

Many people with chronic illnesses will tell you that friends, family, and even strangers have helped them along their way. Six of my friends, as well as my husband, my mother, and my oldest daughter stepped forward to offer me a kidney. My husband was refused by the transplant center because of hints of former Hepatitis B in his blood, and my mother was refused because of her age. My eventual donor was my oldest daughter.

7. Research hospitals/interview surgeons.

> (CHS - Organ Transplant – Choosing an Organ Transplant Center; Graft and Survival Rates)

Here are the questions that I researched before narrowing my choices:
- How many kidney transplants had the center done?
- How many living-related transplants had the center done?
- How did the center's survival (donor, recipient, graft) rates stack up against those of other centers?

- Will the surgeon take the time to talk to you about the operation well ahead of the date of surgery?
- Will the anesthesiologist talk to you about options?
- Will your insurance pay for an out-of-state transplant center (look for "centers of excellence" clauses in your policy)?

I answered all of these questions by looking at large books of published statistics. You can answer them on Colorado HealthSite. I found three transplant centers — all out of state — that ranked equally high on the first three of these questions. I made my final choice by calling each center, telling them that I was considering coming there for a kidney transplant, and asking to speak to a transplant surgeon. Only one transplant center surgeon called me back, Dr. Arthur Matas from the University of Minnesota. That's where I had my transplant done.

8. Go forward after setbacks .

You can read my story on CHS in which I detail setbacks that I faced.

Setbacks are not unexpected when they occur in connection with a serious illness and surgery. We call them unexpected here because patients usually don't want to think about the possibility of things going wrong after they "are fixed."

9. Long-term survival

Long-term survival for people with chronic illnesses has its own set of challenges. As a result of immune suppression, transplant recipients face increased probabilities for cancer, bone disease, diabetes, heart disease, chronic rejection, and less than perfect kidney function. Those with other chronic illnesses face other challenges. One thing we all have in common, however, is the need to find whatever support we can — friends, family, meditation, spiritual faith, visualization, music, massage, etc. — to help us live with as much energy and joy as we can. We deal with this challenge in the next chapter.

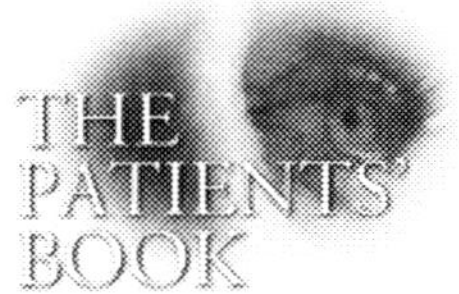

CHAPTER 6

The Acute Phase

After much red tape, reams of paperwork and questions, you enter a hospital — in hopes of a cure, a cessation or reduction of pain and/or a somewhat normal life again You're given a skimpy gown so that your backside is exposed. You're put in a room with a stranger who may moan all night, curse and/or die right there. At the very least, he may want to watch soap operas all day instead of the baseball game. The food? It's usually beige and bland.

While you fade in and out of anesthesia or pain medication, you'll hear the chattering of nurses and foreign clanging sounds from down the hall. Light will always be coming from the doorway. Nurses and doctors of varying stations, educational backgrounds, social skills and competence, will come in your room at all hours, introduce themselves quickly, using unfamiliar titles. Then they will usually do something painful to you - draw blood, give you a shot, move you around. Sometimes they'll put you in a wheelchair, steer you down the hall in your skimpy gown, park you by a door and go away. People with clothes on get to look at you. After a while, someone will do an x-ray or a test, then wheel you back and plunk you in bed. These people will have your chart, which will probably go along with you to x-ray, ultrasound, etc. In most hospitals, however, you will not be able to see your chart.

Sandy's story:

When I was in the hospital to have my hips replaced, various doctors, med students, nurses, and technicians all had access to my chart. When I tried to look at my own records, however, the chart was pulled away from me. One technician who allowed me to look at my chart was reprimanded by a nurse. **It seemed that my privacy was protected only when I was the one trying to see my confidential health records.**

You almost never get to shower or wash your hair and nurses don't have time to "fix you up" anymore. People will visit you without your permission. They come in the door and sit down and start talking. You may get phone calls from well-meaning friends and co-workers. You lose control of your privacy. Anyone can walk in and see you disheveled, snoring, in pain or whatever other unattractive condition that you usually keep to yourself.

The patient is left in a state of confusion. When will the doctor be by? Who knows? What did the tests show? Am I in danger right now? When will I get out? Ask one person and she will respond that you need to talk to someone else.

The above scenario pales when you begin to talk about an operation, the time when you will lose consciousness and give your entire being over to men and women you hope will be paying attention to what they're doing, not joke too loudly in the operating room, make their cuts and their decisions like they were operating on their own mother. It involves total helplessness, many (often unknown) drugs, odd side effects and sometimes much pain and discomfort. Knowing more about the experience will give you some sense of control back.

The most important step: Get a "buddy." Here is our description of the buddy system.

What is the buddy system?

The buddy system is a support team that will help you through both the acute phase and the on-going chronic phase of your illness. The team consists of a group of people who agree to walk all or part of the way with you. The members of your team may or may not know each other and may or may not live near you. They may include:
- a spouse or significant other,
- family members,
- neighbors,
- personal friends,
- office friends,
- established groups such as a book club,
- church or other religious or spiritual group,
- individuals or groups concerned with the same illness on the Web.

The members of your support team will certainly have different strengths and talents. Here are the kinds of talents you should include in your team:
- Someone you can trust enough to tell not only your fears about your illness, but also what questions you are afraid to ask your doctor
- Someone with a good sense of humor
- Someone who is naturally compassionate and empathetic
- Someone who is very assertive and strong when dealing with medical personnel

- Someone who is knowledgeable about the Internet and can help you educate yourself about your illness

It is unlikely that you will find these very different talents in one person and that is why we think you will need a team.

Who needs a buddy?

We know some patients who say they don't want or need a buddy. Here are the typical reasons they give:

- Asking for help is like whining and I don't want to be seen as a whiner (usually a woman).
- I am strong enough to take care of myself in any situation (usually a male).
- I am smart enough to understand what is best for me without help from others (usually a person with a graduate degree).
- I trust my doctor to do the right thing for me (all of us).

Are these people right? Well, yes and no. Those who fall into the first two categories above are worried about how they will be perceived by others. Their fears are not groundless. You may indeed be viewed as a whiner if you admit that you are frightened and need some help. Let us remind you of Sandy's story:

> *... I told my nephrologist that I was scared, that I didn't want to go on dialysis and face a life of being tied to a machine with at best a three-year life span. Here is how he answered me (honest!): "Oh whine, whine, whine — it is always the women and it is always late in the day." ...*

It is also true that some may view you as weak if you admit that you can't take care of yourself alone.

Those who fall into the latter two categories probably don't see themselves as worried about how they are perceived by others. Instead, they just trust that they will find their way through with their own "smarts" and with their trusted doctor. Can they? We know from talking to patients that even those with many degrees (even degrees in health care fields) are just as frightened as the least educated among us to ask questions of our doctors. We were struck by a recent article in the NY Times detailing the conflicts of interest when doctors receive payments from pharmaceutical companies to recruit patients for drug trials. Here is a quote from a health care economist at Princeton University who participated in such a trial, because he feared annoying his doctor and had no idea that money was involved. *"The physician has enormous power over you. You want to keep his favor. If you say no, you'll worry that he (your physician) may not like you."*

A buddy can give you strength, courage, be your advocate and make you laugh

There is nothing wrong with any of the reasons that we give for not needing a buddy. None of us wants to become a whiner and none of us wants to be viewed as weak or medically dumb. All of us must find a way to work with and trust our doctors. The problem is that we must also resolve to put ourselves and our own health as our highest priority. Sometimes, that means asking questions that make our doctors uncomfortable or even angry, causing us to lose our resolve. This is where our buddy can take over.

What a buddy can do for you

The benefits of a buddy are virtually endless. He or she can:
- Accompany you to your doctor's appointment and ask the questions you are too scared to ask or forget to ask because of the stress you feel.
- Be a sounding board for you to discuss treatment options and help you choose among those options in an objective and logical manner.
- Give you the strength and courage to keep going when you feel overwhelmed by your illness.
- Make you laugh.
- Motivate you to keep trying to get help when your doctor has decided that you don't have a real illness.
- Motivate you to walk or exercise in other ways when you are too depressed or have too much pain to get out of your house or apartment.
- Be your advocate in the hospital to make sure that you are not given the wrong medications and are treated with dignity by your nurses and doctors.
- Help you find the medical information you need to understand your illness and the range of treatments that are available.

Choosing a buddy

Have a conversation with the buddy beforehand, even if you think you know him or her well, and explain your concept of an advocate - his/her role is not to "go along" with whatever happens, but to question and be assertive for you if need be.

Jenny's story:

Jenny made sure to have a friend with her during an operation. But she began to have problems with pain and with her medications. She asked her friend to talk with the doctors; her friend returned and told her "Don't worry. The doctors said everything is just fine."

This is NOT the kind of person you need to help you through this experience.

Your friend should also be someone you're entirely comfortable with, because often you're not going to feel like entertaining him. A good friend will bring a book, etc., and be able to sit quietly with you. Doctors and nurses may disagree with this concept, but we believe, given recent cutbacks and changes in our health care system, having a buddy with you is essential. At the very least, your buddy can help you be more comfortable, bring you water and ice or other items you might need, help you walk around. At the most, he can save your life.

Age doesn't matter. Twenty-two year old Carrie was a great advocate for her brother.

Carrie's story:

In March 1999, my brother Mark was thrown from a Range Rover. The Rover flipped and landed on him, crushing his body. He was flown by helicopter to a medical center in New Jersey. He had a broken neck, back, left leg, jaw, and collar bone. The doctors performed surgery on his neck, using bone grafts from his hip. Further procedures repaired his jaw and leg. Our family was devastated by the tragedy. The instant I learned about the accident, I flew in from my college in Colorado. Over the next few weeks, I spent many hours at the hospital. By the second or third day, I became quite familiar with the routine. Mark was fed at certain times, given high doses of morphine, had his teeth brushed, bandages changed – all on a schedule. Part of the routine involved moving him into something called an orthopedic chair. The chair was designed to prevent his lungs from stagnating, which could cause pneumonia. On one particular occasion when Mark was to be moved into the chair, the floor was understaffed and so the nurses called on the four security guards for help. My mother and father, nervous about this, aided the nurses as well. On the count of three, everyone was to lift my brother, using the sheet under him as a stretcher of sorts. No sooner than I heard the word "three," the security guards who were unfamiliar with Mark's injuries, flung him into the orthopedic chair. His head flew back and Mark cried out loudly in pain. My mother screamed also. I ran out of the room to find the orthopedic surgeon, who was walking down the hall. I told him about the accident and the poor way in which the transfer was handled. He did not seem alarmed in the slightest. To make matters worse, Mark's broken leg was heavy and continually caused the chair to fall forward. To correct this, the nurses propped the chair and his leg up with office chairs and a garbage can at one point. The incident left my brother paranoid to be moved; he dreaded that chair.

Mark had IVs in his arms and hands through which morphine was administered, along with other drugs. Whenever a nurse came in with an injection, I would ask what it was they were giving him. One day, a nurse came in with what she said was morphine. She injected it into the IV and left the room. A few minutes passed and another nurse came in with an injection. I asked what it was and he told me "morphine." I told him that Mark had already been given his morphine and asked that he double-check his orders with the head nurse. After a small debate, he left and checked with the head nurse. He came back into the room, said I had been right, and left. Two shots of morphine would have knocked Mark out for quite a while contrary to the doctor's orders which were for Mark to stay active and awake.

These mistakes, which may seem small and insignificant to a medical professional, were extremely upsetting to my family. We were grateful to have each other and the ability to stay with my brother at all times. He was never left alone, one of us was always with him. We were lucky to be able to do that. Our constant presence allowed us to take care of my brother and to catch those "little" mistakes that would have otherwise gone unnoticed.

Sometimes parents need to be reminded to suppress their own fears in order to be a good advocate for their son or daughter.

Patricia recounts her conversation with a stranger she met on a plane on her way to her son's house after he was diagnosed with a rare form of cancer:

Don was in his third year of medical school. He had always been my radiant and strong boy, never even prone to colds. Don called one night with the news that he had cancer. It was a rare kind and the outcome was not predictable. I flew to be with him and his wife. On the plane, I was a wreck, shaking and sometimes crying. The man next to me asked me what was wrong and I told him. After he listened to my story, we talked for quite a while. Before we got off the plane, he looked at me sternly and said: 'You have to pull yourself together. You're an intelligent and rational person and your son is going to NEED you'. It was important for me that he said that. For a while I could put aside my terror and fear and turn to my son to be whatever help I could.

Preparing for the hospital

Before you go to the hospital, talk to your doctor and the anesthesiologist. Patients usually don't know when (or if) they'll see the doctors. Ask yours if he/she will be in charge of your care in the hospital. Will she make regular visits to you? How often? What time of day? At least a week before an operation, talk to the surgeon (if you can't do that, reconsider the operation). Find out how often he's performed this operation. Ask him about the possibility of complications, infections. Sometimes big name doctors only do part of the operation - ask if your surgeon plans to do the whole thing. Talk with the anesthesiologist before the operation (not the night before when you're tired and scared). Be sure he knows your history. Ask what kind of anesthesia he will be giving you. Find out if he will be with you the whole time.

If you're going to need blood, think about having it drawn ahead of time, so you'll get your own blood, or blood donated from friends or family. Talk to your surgeon about what pain control methods will be used after the operation. Some doctors want you to have shots when you begin to feel pain; others approve a self-medicating pump. After an operation is not the time to be brave - if you stay in pain and let it get out of control, your mental and emotional outlook is not going to be good. Adequate medication for pain is still controversial among many physicians.

The authors of a study on elderly cancer patients stated that "pain is one of cancer's most frequent and disturbing symptoms" despite the fact that the appropriate use of pain medications "can relieve pain in more than 90% of cases." Many reasons were given for the failure to give patients adequate pain medication - inadequate staff to provide and monitor frequent pain administration, and the inadequate knowledge and failure of many physicians to use analgesic agents aggressively, and the unwillingness of patients to report pain because of "fear that reporting pain will take physician time away from the treatment of their cancer." The authors of the study were very clear about their position: "Failure to prevent and/or treat pain effectively at virtually all times is no longer acceptable and should be considered (an indicator) of poor quality of medical care."

Choosing a hospital

Pay attention to the choice of hospital. Be sure it's approved by JCAHO, the Joint Commission of Accreditation of Healthcare Organizations (which performs most inspections of hospitals) or the group that accredits osteopathic hospitals.

If you know a nurse, ask him or her which hospital he or she would go to. If any friends have been in a hospital recently (and that's important, because the operation of a hospital can change quickly), find out their experience.

You can also go to the hospital and check it out. Is it crowded? Is it clean? Are people on the staff helpful? Does the air smell fresh? Do the patients have enough personal space? Do the patients each have water pitchers with glasses? Do staff members seem respectful of patients? Is the hospital a teaching facility (in a teaching hospital, medical personnel will be in your room often, discussing your case, and your care will mostly be done by residents and interns under the direction of a doctor) or a private hospital? Some people prefer a teaching hospital because it's often the center of a health complex where the students are exposed to the latest medical developments and studies and often research is on the cutting edge. Others find the environment very intrusive.

What hospitals are like

You need to know the rules and rhythms of a hospital, which can be the most alien of places. The more you know, the more comfortable (emotionally) you'll be.

In the Door:

If your admission is not an emergency, you'll be asked to bring papers such as insurance card, health records, advanced medical directive (instructions as to what others should do medically, if you're not able to respond…this may include a living will), durable power of attorney, etc. You'll be asked to sign a consent form. You should ask questions related to your condition - if they find X, what are they likely to do?

- Things to bring. Don't wear your contacts; bring glasses. Bring less than $5 and no valuables. Bring a few toilet items (brush and comb, emery board, etc.), a TV guide, a book or some magazines, family pictures, a cheap watch. Don't forget to write down the names and phone numbers of people you may need or want to call during your hospital stay - neighbors who are taking care of your house, someone to pick you up, your doctor's number, etc. Ask your doctor about bringing medications you regularly take. Bring your pillow from home; ask about bringing your own pajamas.
- Roommate or not? They can be irritating. On the other hand, roommates can be very comforting, especially if that person has a condition similar to yours.

In Your Room:

Various medical people will come in and introduce themselves. Ones to pay the most attention to are the RNs (registered nurses), who will probably be in charge of the floor, and the Licensed Practical Nurses (LPNs) or Certified Nurse Assistants (CNAs). Someone will take your pulse and temperature and do an assessment. Someone should explain about the phone, call button, the television, when meals are served and what your choices are. You need to tell someone (and maybe several people) about any allergies you have to medicine or food. Make sure your allergies are posted on your chart and near your bed. You must tell them about medications you are taking now.

Surgery and ICU (Intensive Care Unit):

Usually you won't see the surgery room; you will have been given something to make you sleep before that. Often, you'll wake up back in your room. If you do wake up in Intensive Care, you're likely to see wires, tubes, large equipment, bright lights and medical personnel bustling around - it can look scary. They will be checking your vital signs often, and perhaps doing tests (taking blood, etc.).

Taking care of yourself:

Many patients fear that if they complain or use the call button too frequently or ask for more pain medication, they'll be labeled "problem patients" by the nurses - and they'll be ignored by these all-important people who run the hospitals. Be aware that even though you are still in pain, most doctors and nurses want you to be as active as you can and start to take responsibility for your care almost immediately. That doesn't mean you shouldn't call a nurse when you're in pain or need something you can't handle yourself. If you feel that your nurse is waiting too long or not treating you properly, talk to him/her. If that doesn't work, ask to see the Charge Nurse. The next person up the chain of command is the Nursing Supervisor. Some hospitals have a Patient Representative you can talk with. Complaining is a job you may want to turn over to your "buddy."

Keep a notepad by your bed and jot down questions so that you'll remember them when the doctor comes in. Doctors and nurses spent many years learning to speak their own language - but when they're talking to you, ask them to speak in language you can understand. Say you'd like for them to be honest and let you know exactly what's going on. Repeat if necessary: "I don't understand what you just said; please put it in terms I can understand."

Some patients feel more comfortable in their own clothes - check the hospital policy. The short cotton gown is efficient when many tests need to be done. For a little more privacy, put one gown on frontward and one on backwards.

Keep your wits. Even in this difficult time, don't turn yourself over anymore than necessary to your doctors or hospital. Because you may be weak, in pain and dazed, talk to your buddy several times a day to discuss what's going on and get her to give you feedback. Be straightforward in expressing your concerns.

Pay attention to the drugs you're given. Know what you're going to get (ask the doctor), what it looks like and how many times a day. If you're not given what you expect, speak up.

If you're offered food before an operation, or a diet you suspect is wrong, speak up. If you're given a sleeping pill and think you don't need it, don't take it. You have the right to refuse medication. Especially in a teaching hospital, if you believe your blood is being drawn too many times, speak to the doctor.

Going home:

Even when you know it's the day you're supposed to leave, medical personnel can be maddeningly vague about exactly when. Often, it's because they can't release you until the doctor gives an approval, and they don't know when the doctor will be there.

Don't let anyone rush you out of the hospital. If you're feeling nauseated, be sure and tell someone and get medication - or don't leave. Write down the instructions for what you're supposed to do at home - medicines, exercises, diet, rest, having sexual relations, going back to work, driving a car. Don't even think you'll remember everything! Does the doctor have a treatment plan? Go over it with her. If she doesn't give you one, ask for guidance. When will you see the doctor again? Have you made a follow-up appointment? Who do you call if something goes wrong? If you need special equipment, has someone seen to that? Have you been given special stockings commonly used after surgery to protect against blood clots? Ask the doctor how you should feel - in a few days, in a week. In certain cases, it might help you to talk to someone else who has had the same procedure. Your doctor could give you some phone numbers.

Once home, it's still important to have a buddy.

Sally stunned her friends when she had a heart attack. She was fit, ate a good diet, but had a genetic history of heart disease. Her husband took his role of buddy seriously. After she had emergency surgery, he discouraged people from visiting in the hospital because she was so tired and in a lot of pain. When she got home, he again guarded her wellbeing by being sure nobody visited too long. Sally said "I probably wouldn't have said no to visits sometimes, but he did it for me."

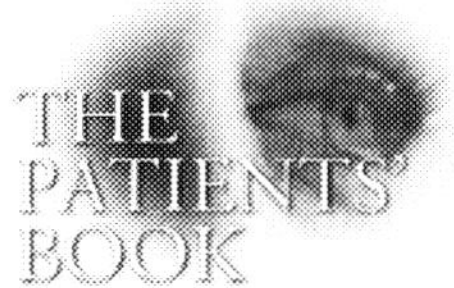

Chapter 7

Chronic Illnesses:
Preparing for the Long Haul

A TV ad for a painkiller shows the pages of a calendar flying away. "Don't you wish you could go back to the time before you had arthritis?" a voice asks.

Anyone with a chronic illness will feel a pang while watching that. Even though symptoms may have been present for quite a while, it seems almost as if one day you're a whole, healthy, vigorous person (with a few aches and pains), and the next day you're the name of a disease: M.S., heart disease, cancer, a dialysis patient. Of course some people have no symptoms or pain at all; often cancer patients feel fine until they're diagnosed and then begin treatment. Automatically your world becomes smaller. You're focused on the illness and your life almost becomes the disease.

It's a healthy reaction, at least for a while. Even if you were in initial denial (a stage almost everyone goes through), you now have a diagnosis, a name to put on your pain. You turn inward and feel what's going on; you notice where the aches are and when they happen. You reach out to others who have the same problem. You read and research the subject.

You may become depressed. You desperately want to turn those pages back to when you could run, bike, ski and play - or perhaps just breathe without pain — with abandon, without hesitation. You're heard the expression that life isn't fair and now you're experiencing that. Some well-meaning person will point out someone in a wheelchair or someone who's had a heart transplant, telling you how lucky you are not to be in that person's situation. The comparison doesn't help. You've got a problem; the main thought is that your real and normal life is over and will never be the same. You may face death, have your life brutally shortened or at least have to live with disabilities the rest of your days.

A positive attitude and spirit
of optimism can increase the quality
and duration of your life

The courage and determination that got you through the acute part of your illness may be flagging at the prospect that you have to live with this disability the rest of your life. Sometimes it takes a word from someone else to "inspire" you.

Sandy's story:
After my transplant I went into rejection and had to return to the hospital for anti-rejection treatment. That treatment began with 500 mg of solumedrol administered intravenously and then went on to a drug called OKT3, which was also administered intravenously. Because my veins are small, each intravenous drug required at least 2 and some-

times 3–4 attempts before successful. The 11 days of OKT3 sent me into delirium, caused me to vomit continuously and to lose my hearing.

At one point I refused an intravenous drug, saying I would rather die than have anything more put into my veins. The young Indian doctor who was sent to administer the drug looked at me disapprovingly and said: "Pull yourself together, you have a long row to hoe and you have a duty to fight for this kidney, which is a precious gift." Embarrassed and admonished, I sat still for the intravenous drug.

If you have a chronic illness, you need information and education. You need facts about the illness, treatment options, descriptions of medications (including side effects and interactions with other drugs) and up-to-date information about clinical studies and medical research that may impact you.

Equally important are management skills, emotional support and your outlook on life. You may have heard the expression "Attitude is all." When you can't walk or have trouble breathing, you may scoff at any attitude besides despair. But so many studies have shown a positive attitude and a spirit of optimism can increase the quality - and duration - of your life. If that's not your natural bent, it's certainly something to point yourself toward.

The psychological part

Where are the doctors when we need them? Like most of us, they'd like to identify a problem, fix it and then be proud of what a good job they did. This can't happen with most chronic situations. There's talk of "treatment plans," but few patients ever see them.

When you're in the "not sick, not cured" category, it's sometimes hard to get the medical community to pay attention to you. You may feel invisible. In an essay about patients on dialysis ("The

Marginal Man") author Melanie K. Landsman tells what it's like to live in the never-never land of a severe chronic illness. She explains:

The person with chronic renal disease will have at least one crisis and find himself "dependent, passive and in need of substantial medical attention." At this point, he is a "patient" and he's "sick" and "accepted as free from normal functioning." Then he may be stabilized by dialysis. His psychological problem "is created by the contradiction that he feels better, but that he is not and cannot be cured." He is getting a treatment, but no cure. He is not dying nor is he returned to society "healed." The dialysis patient is told to go lead a normal life, but to follow a strict regime of food and fluids. He can return to work, but shouldn't miss any of his treatments. He is advised not to fixate on his illness and treatment, but also told he should expect to feel lethargic and, by the way, he may be impotent. It's limbo, it's confusing, it's a feeling of being marginalized.

Can't shake hands

Part of the problem is that many of us don't look sick. Those with severe arthritis can radiate health, but try to shake hands with them and it knocks them to the floor. Persons with fibromyalgia may look fine, but can be aching from head to toe. People with chronic illnesses can feel relatively fine one day and awful the next - with no change in how they look. Often they couldn't get a diagnosis from a doctor (and they may have gone to quite a few) and sometimes they heard phrases that sounded like "it's all in your head."

Hugh said, "After I was first diagnosed with MS it bothered me when people said I looked good. There seemed to be an implication that I was malingering or exaggerating."

Clela said, "I can't tell you how many times I wished my migraine headaches and fibromyalgia would manifest into some visible defect so people could see how much I hurt."

Nobody wants to be labeled a complainer or a whiner. But sometimes you desperately want someone to understand that you are in pain, that there is a problem and you're dealing with it the best you can. The specter of having some kind of pain the rest of your life, or having to take a myriad of pills, do endless exercises or change your diet, is not pleasant. Grimmer still is the idea that you may have good days and bad, but your condition will gradually get worse. "I don't ever want to have a chronic illness," one nurse told us. "I just want to keel over one day." He went on to say that every nurse he knew agreed with him. "One nurse swears she has 'do not resuscitate' tattooed on her chest."

Guilt? Blame?

Part of the depression and pain of a chronic condition comes from the belief that you brought it on yourself. You could spend a lot of time wishing away poor nutrition, sedentary habits, use of tobacco or drugs or alcohol. You may wish you had better genes and a better upbringing. All that is beside the point. You have a long-term problem to deal with and guilt isn't going to help. You may feel blamed by some doctors or medical personnel. They're trained to cure you - and chronic patients, or those diagnosed with a terminal disease, don't fall into that category. Getting help with your chronic illness may be much harder than having a doctor focus on an acute problem that he/she can solve and pronounce you cured (or at least much better). And while it may be fairly easy to rally friends and family for an illness of short duration, it's quite another thing to look at long-term care.

So, there's a lot to deal with, but you don't have to do it all at once. This is about the quality of life for the rest of your life. Break it down into pieces you can manage and get started.

Your own treatment plan: some control

If your doctor doesn't provide a long-term plan for your condition, you should make one for yourself (and/or you can elaborate on the one given you). With the knowledge you have and the research tools you are now familiar with, you are equipped. And maybe your doctor will even agree with it.

Here are some initial questions to answer:
- What type of immediate care do I need?
- What about the long term? What kind of help will I need?
- Am I on top of insurance issues or do I need to get help with them?
- What kind of exercise should I be doing to maintain the best health?
- Are there things I absolutely should not be doing?
- What's the best food plan for my condition?
- How can I still have a support network without wearing out my friends?
- How can I develop a good long term working partnership with my doctors?
- Should I be taking a drug for this condition?
- Are the drugs I'm taking helpful, working, sufficient?

Treatment plan examples:

Preparing for your future

Diane's story:

Because I had time to plan before my hip replacement, I was able to be fairly organized. I decided to sell the bungalow I lived in; it had stairs and was going to need a lot of upkeep and yard work in the future (I wasn't interested in spending time or energy on that). I moved to a condo, where my unit was on one floor and easy to clean. Sunlight streamed in from two sides. The kitchen was arranged with an island, making cooking easy when I was on crutches. The condo had a heated pool, hot tub, exercise room and nearby neighbors, a "feature" that made me feel more secure.

Before the operation, I removed obstacles (throw rugs, etc.) and put anything I would need for the next couple of months on shelves so I wouldn't have to bend over or reach down. I stacked up slip-on clothing.

I set up a "command center" – an easy chair in the den, with a phone, TV, stack of magazines and books, list of important phone numbers, TV remote control. I made sure there was enough space in several rooms for me to exercise, something I would start the day I came home. Probably most important, I did exercises daily for weeks before the operation; this was a command from the surgeon.

Someone suggested I get a gardening apron. This was indispensable for the six weeks I was on crutches. The nine little apron pockets were perfect for glasses, a Coke, a cell phone, pen, etc. I got a bike bag for the walker I also used. An upstairs neighbor volunteered to stop by my condo every morning at 10, escort me to the pool and swim with me.

My daughter stayed with me for almost a week when I got out of the hospital. She was great company, but after the first couple of days, I wanted to be up and cooking and moving around as much as possible. I exercised, swam and read my instructions religiously, being careful not to break any of the new hip "rules." I found someone to come and clean once a week, a huge help because I dropped things all the time. The first Saturday I was home, I invited friends over to a brunch – I asked them to bring food and I would have the coffee. They thought I was crazy but I loved having the company (and I kept the leftovers!). Friends often stopped by and brought lunch. Several good friends brought groceries periodically; a man in my building would visit daily, and would take the trash out for me. That was for the short term – a period of recuperation that lasted about two months (although I went back to work after a month).

For the long run, I knew I should keep my weight down and exercise. I think regular exercise is the best treatment for arthritis. After a while, I could walk to and from work (about 2 1/2 miles round trip), use the treadmill and other machines and swim. In good weather, I bike.

For days when pain seems ever present, I try to stay warm. I sleep on a mattress pad with magnets, which I believe helps the pain and problems with sleeping. I listen to music that lifts me up or I get absorbed in studying a subject I love. And it always helps to tell someone special that "I hurt all over" and get a long hug – maybe the best medicine of all.

Although the doctor said I would need the other hip replaced within ten years, I'll try to avoid that by doing all the healthy things I can and buying some time until they come up with something better. I don't need a support group, but I do subscribe to Arthritis Today and watch Colorado HealthSite for new developments

Developing a Long-Term Partnership with your Doctor

Robert's Story:

I am 63 years old. I take several drugs for my arthritis. I also exercise every day and almost always eat a healthy diet. I don't smoke and drink very seldom. I have no family history of heart disease. So, I was surprised when I began one evening to have a pounding feeling in my chest. The feeling lasted about 4 hours and the next morning I was short of breath. I ignored the first episode, but decided to take action when the second episode occurred. My doctor put me on a heart monitor that I was to wear for two weeks. After 3 days, my doctor called and said I could return the monitor because the monitor had already recorded two episodes of atrial fibrillation.

She sent me to have a complete heart work up – echocardiogram and cardiolite stress test. Then, she sent me to a heart specialist, Doctor Y, who talked to me about the test results. Here is what he said: my heart was structurally sound. The stress test showed excellent exercise tolerance and the blood flow during exercise was also excellent. I attempted to ask questions about the causes of my atrial fibrillation, the possible triggers, and the impact of changes in diet. The doctor was visibly annoyed at my questions and finally said that we only had a short time and he was an expert and couldn't have his patients second guessing him. There was a standard treatment protocol for idiopathic atrial fibrillation (unrelated to underlying heart disease). The standard treat-

ment protocol was the use of a calcium channel blocker, followed by Coumadin if my episodes increased in duration or frequency.

When I got home, I called my gateway doctor and said I could not work with Dr. Y because he was uncomfortable with patient partnership and that I wanted a referral to another doctor in the same group. She agreed. I told the next heart specialist I visited that I worked best in a partnership and asked if he was comfortable with that. He said he was. We talked about some possible triggers of atrial fibrillation (coffee, wine, chocolate) and he said that the standard treatment protocol for someone like me was a calcium channel blocker. I told him I didn't want to take another drug and asked if I was putting my life at risk by refusing that treatment. He said no and we parted with an agreement to keep in touch if my symptoms got worse.

All of us could learn a valuable lesson from Robert's experience. The best of modern medicine allowed him and his doctors to discover that, although he did have atrial fibrillation, he had no underlying heart disease. Instead of getting angry at his first heart specialist, Robert simply asked for another referral. His understanding gateway doctor made an appointment for him with another heart specialist. Robert refused the standard treatment, but did so in a way that assured him he wasn't taking a risk and allowed him to continue building a good partnership with a specialist who might be needed in the future.

Some Comforting Things to Consider

Surely, we all ought to think about what comforts us, what makes us feel the best. But with the hurried pace of life most of us live, we usually don't even get enough sleep. When you have a chronic illness, one that practically sits in your lap to remind you that you're in pain or disabled, we believe it's necessary to counteract that pain (emotional and physical) with large and small joys and comforts.

Once again, you need to turn inward, relax, be in a quiet spot and get to know yourself a little better. You may even want to remember what made you happy as a child. What we're going for always is a sense of control - and being able to make yourself feel better, more optimistic and happier will certainly do that.

WARM WATER: A very warm tub of water (or a real hot tub if you're lucky) can help erase, for the moment, all kinds of aches and pains. The buoyancy you experience can last beyond the tub. Often we're tensed for pain and a bath can reduce that tension.

HOT TEA, COCOA: Warming your insides with something you enjoy can be a ritual that signals some pampering to your body. You almost have to sit down to drink it and a short rest plus some hot tea may be the luxury you need.

WARM CLOTHING: A pair of down booties for feet that ache, a cotton robe against sensitive skin, flannel clothing - all can support your sense of well being. For people with many illnesses, being cold is going to make them feel worse. Is there a cozy afghan nearby that you can throw over you?

Music: If it's a soaring aria, a subtle violin concerto, or down-and-dirty rock 'n' roll - listen and see if you feel better when you hear it. People who can hardly walk have been known to dance a little in the privacy of their homes, and feel ten times better when they're through. You might like inspirational or jazz - try it out.

Massage: This is often considered an expense that's hard to justify - but those who have found relief from pain will praise massage to the heavens. In a recent issue of Psychology Today (March/April 1999, p. 23), several presentations at the American Massage Therapy Association were cited. One showed that one group of cancer patients who got a massage reported less pain and stress than the control group. "Massage also seems to rev up the immune system in times of fatigue and anxiety."

Loving Touch: If you have a mate, ask for long hugs, a loving arm around you. Let friends know you like to be hugged. It's healing.

Scents: Aromatherapy has become quite popular and you can find an array of scents at health food stores. One way to begin is to just choose a candle that smells good to you, that triggers a good memory or makes you feel happier. Experiment, but watch out for allergies.

Comfort Foods: We know a woman who thinks chicken liver is a comfort food — that's what her mother used to feed her when she was sick. Unfortunately, most of us would like to leap into the nearest chocolate cake for comfort. Cake or rice pudding all day long probably isn't a great idea, but it shouldn't hurt you every once in a while. We often deprive ourselves of carbohydrates while dieting, but breads, cereal, etc. can be very comforting and they're good for you. Read up on nutrition and find what foods are most healing. And don't forget chicken soup!

DIVERSIONS: One man we know who has almost constant pain will go on a marathon movie binge when he's feeling especially bad. It takes his mind off his body. Whatever works; try movies, videos, games with friends, the Internet, books or audio books. It's been said that you need to find something in your life that's as absorbing as your pain. Finding out what that is, in itself, may prove a wonderful distraction.

WATER EXERCISE: Exercising in warm water can be wonderfully comforting to those with aching joints and muscles. In situations where routine exercise is encouraged (and it almost always is), this is a way to do it with minimal pain. Even those not comfortable with swimming can often relax when they have a mask and snorkel on, and can paddle around a pool for a long time.

LOOKING YOUR BEST: If you look in the mirror at your bedraggled self, hair askew and face pale, there's a good chance it will make you feel worse. Put on your best face; comfortable, clean and attractive clothes (well, at least a bright jogging suit), get a good haircut, manicure and pedicure (or ask a friend), brush your hair, shave and shower. Try to smile and be upbeat, even if you don't always feel that way.

FRIENDS: Sometimes people who care about you don't know what to do when you're sick. You need to decide how much company you want, how much energy you have to be with people, how much help you need and what you can ask others to do without wearing out your friendships. You might ask a friend to pick up some dinner and share it with you. Another might be happy to take you for a drive, or to the store. Be with people who give you energy. Keep your distance from those who sap your energy - even if they're family. Be sure you're asking your friends questions about their lives, not always talking about your illness. And when you do talk about your illness, it's okay to tell that person you just want to talk, that you'd rather not have advice right now.

BEAUTIFUL SURROUNDINGS: If it's not beautiful where you spend most of your time, get help in making your environment peaceful and lovely. If you have to sit and look at a gray wall or wiring overhead or have no window and no sunlight, it can have a subconscious effect on your attitude. It doesn't have to be expensive and might just involve bringing a comfortable chair near the window so you can look out at the birds.

HELPING OTHERS: It's a cliche, but true for many. If you can help others, it means you're not quite so helpless. It can also be healing to help someone with your same condition.

GETTING OUTDOORS: Your mother was right: Go play outdoors. If you can walk or hike in the outdoors, or even wheel in a wheelchair, chances are you're going to come inside feeling better. If you're in a routine of staying inside, make the effort to get out.

INTELLECTUAL CHALLENGES: Pick up a crossword puzzle, convince someone to play Scrabble with you or read some history, biography, or fiction. When you're making demands on your brain, there's less room for thinking about your pain.

VISUALIZATION: Some people find great help is visualizing their bodies healing, in seeing with their mind's eye what they can do in the future. Others relieve stress by visualizing their favorite place (real or dream), a scene they can put themselves in and feel peaceful and happy. Plenty of books and tapes can help you with this practice.

MEDITATION: If your idea of meditation is sitting very still and thinking of "nothing," you might investigate a little further. One definition of meditation is doing something (jogging, martial arts, ballet) that completely distracts you from your problems. And there's still the type of meditation where you learn to relax through deep breathing and sometimes saying a mantra. We often read medical studies that confirm that meditation is a great stress reliever.

SPIRITUALITY: Religion, higher power, faith, whatever you want to call it - can give hope and comfort to those in pain. Find your own path.

HUMOR: Perhaps this should be first on the list, not last. A most famous example of how much help laughter can be is found in *Anatomy of my Illness*, a book by Norman Cousins. Faced with a terminal diagnosis, he decided to cure himself with humor and Vitamin C. Rent some funny movies, have some belly laughs and forget yourself for a while.

FILL IN YOUR OWN: What makes you feel comforted? More alive? Less pain? Think of this as your job - take it seriously.

Mobilize your support team

For many of us, asking for help is one of the hardest things we can ever do. We may hesitate to impose on someone's time and energy, even our best friend or a close family member. But, the truth is, it's almost always gratifying to help someone else. It makes us feel important, needed and useful.

If you have a chronic illness, a support system is crucial. Don't forget to ASK for what you need. You'll need other people too - spread it around so no one gets weary of listening, etc. You may come out of this experience with more and closer friends that you had before.

Mary's story:

When I was diagnosed with cancer of the bone, all the people in my office organized to feed me. They put a list out and signed up every night for the first month; after that it was three times a week. They brought wonderful food - sometimes I could eat it and sometimes I couldn't. But it was always a treat to have them walk through the door with a joke and a hug and news about what was going on. They sent me cards, books, flowers and a lot of email.

People don't always volunteer to do something like this because they don't know you need it. If you're able to have company, you could call friends you haven't been able to spend time with in a long time, tell them what's going on and ask: "Could you bring lunch or dinner over and visit?" You'll get very few no's.

Back to mother web

Two things that may raise your spirits and/or comfort level will be connecting with others who have your same problem and being sure you're on top of the latest development in your illness and treatments for it.

Friends and medical buddies can be physically close at hand or close through the Internet. Clela was very skeptical about going on the Internet to find a "buddy." "It's not in my nature to do that," she said. "But a friend kept insisting, so I finally put my name and email out there in the Pen Pals section of Colorado HealthSite."

She and the friend she found, a woman named Judith who lives in Canada, have been corresponding for almost a year. They usually email each other two or three times a week. Both women have fibromyalgia, along with other health problems. The letters are remarkable for their honesty, insight, support of each other and above all, some dry, hilarious commentary on just about everything. As the correspondence progressed, they talked about their families, their work or lack of it, books they've read, politics in each country. They always exchange news about how they were feeling ("even my eyelids hurt") and any tidbits of information on treatment or drugs ("have you tried…..?"). When one person is feeling good, the letters are like those between happy sisters or best friends; when one is especially down, the comforting, empathetic words are like balm.

"It's hard to tell other people how bad you feel," Clela explained. "You need to share it with someone who has the same problem." She doesn't want people to think of her as a "whiner," and both of them have problems that aren't visible to other people when they're in pain. So they lean on each other and get support. "I get a general uplift, a little boost. It's easier to talk to her and confess

I'm feeling crappy. I feel like I'm whining if I talk to others. With her, and maybe it's the distance, too, I can complain for a few sentences, then go on and talk about other things in life. It's satisfying; you've been able to tell somebody you hurt."

Judith has written Clela about a fairly isolated cabin that she and her husband and daughter go to. "Her cabin sounds so healing to me. I can picture it because she's described it so thoroughly. I love to think about it."

Last summer, when Judith had to go in the hospital, Clela was scared when she didn't receive letters. Finally, Judith's daughter started emailing her until Judith was out of the hospital and could speak for herself. The two women are now plotting a time and place they could get together in person and continue their friendship.

Listen to Tori who entered the Fibromyalgia Forum on Colorado HealthSite soon after she was diagnosed with fibromyalgia syndrome (FMS). She introduced herself as newly diagnosed and then asked a couple of questions. She received many answers from others in the forum and then posted this:

I can't keep thanking everyone individually! But I want everyone who has responded to my post to know that you all have helped me very much! I am feeling emotionally a lot better thanks to all of your responses! Cecil is right, all these responses have encouraged me a great deal and have made a world of difference to my emotional state. I hope I can find the right words for someone else new to the scene as I get adjusted to FMS, as you all have done for me. Shoot, I don't get this many personal phone calls in a week. You all are great! And I love you for your kindness!! Forever grateful. Tori

You can find people to talk to on Colorado HealthSite; you can also ask your doctor for the names of people who have your problem and who might like to talk. Be sure you connect with someone positive.

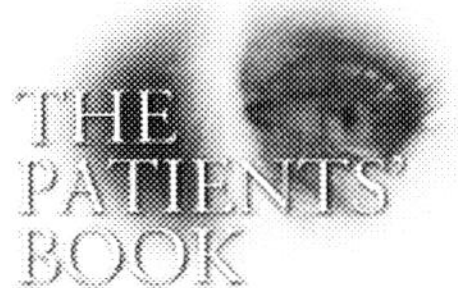

CHAPTER 8

Moving On

In this chapter, we assume that you have received a diagnosis and have finished (for now at least) the acute interventions that you have chosen to accept. Now, you face a life with an ongoing chronic illness and perhaps continuing drug therapy. Some of you will have been told you have months or a few years to live. Still we believe that your work now is to move on - to find meaning, joy, and energy in your new life.

"Moving On" can mean many different things. At first, as we finish with the acute medical intervention phase of our illness, many of us need to talk with other patients who understand what we have gone through. No one else understands in quite the same way what has happened to us. Through patient groups, we get valuable information and support from other patients who have preceded us. For some of us, the need to talk about our illness and its aftermath can become almost an obsession, particularly if our illness has left us with physical or mental limitations and our "cure" is predicted to be short-term. In our view, lots of important work is going on during this period.

We believe, however, that it is important after some period of time to strike out in a new direction so that we don't become our illness.

Here are some ways that people we interviewed have "moved on":

Finding and accepting the gifts that have come as a result of your illness.

Hugh's story:

After a diagnosis of MS, confirmation with a second opinion and acceptance of the reality of having a debilitating, non-fatal, chronic and non-curable disease, the next challenge is to develop the best possible regimen for coping with the disease and moving on to develop a good life in spite of the disease. In my own case, I remember that I received the news of the diagnosis initially with a sense of relief. It was good to know that it wasn't all in my head and that the weird symptoms I had experienced could be explained rationally.

Then came a variety of emotions: denial, anger, regret, guilt, despair, even self-pity. And finally, thank God, acceptance. I slowly became aware, almost by accident, that having MS was not the end of the world and that life was still worth living. At least two things were very fortunate for me: I was lucky to have a loyal, supportive, loving spouse, and my symptoms did not become debilitating until later in life, after I had done most of the things I especially wanted to do.

And so, a number of substitutions took place. My career in law, always before so important, gave way to the pleasures of early retirement. Many things I had not had time for became possible, like reading for pleasure, studying long neglected subjects such as physics and the classics, and listening—really listening—to music. Instead of traveling often, climbing mountains, skiing, running every day and play-

ing handball or tennis almost as often, I learned to play chess, started taking Teaching Company courses and became intensely interested in our Great Books group. Grandchildren, children and friends absorbed more time and physical activities less. Moving on means that I now wonder how I ever had time to work. MS has become more of an irritation than an all-consuming disease. Indeed, I can almost say that MS is a blessing in disguise because it has made me focus on the things in life that are truly important

Ben's story:

If there has been a gift from my cancer it is in the peace I have found in meditation and prayer. In 1994 I trained in The Silva Method, a technique for meditation and visualization, which has become an integral part of my life. Some have been able to resolve their cancer or other illnesses with the power of their mind. I have not found that gift, but I have certainly found a healing and resolution of the anxiety that comes with the knowledge of impending demise. I believe that is a fair trade-off. If I can recommend only one thing to others who may be seriously ill it would be to learn and practice meditation.

Accepting that you have a chronic illness for which there is no cure and few mitigations of symptoms.

Rita's story:

My 50th birthday was a horrible night – that was the first episode with what I learned later was fibromyalgia. I went through a lot of dead ends with doctors and hospitals. Doctors didn't understand. One suggested a brain tumor. Another suggested a psychiatrist – it was so degrading, so accusatory, so demeaning. I would never let someone have that power over me again. If a doctor ever began to go in that direction,

I would stop him and wouldn't deal with him. After finally getting a diagnosis, I decided I needed to make peace with my own pain. I sort of said "Pain, you're part of my body, how am I going to live with you?" I realized I had to go on with my life.

For me, "moving on" literally means moving — I learned that by moving, I was better off, even though it felt better not to move - I really wanted to go to bed and cover my head. But the more intensely I exercise, the better I feel. Maybe endorphins are kicking in.

When I have "episodes," I try to figure out why this time is worse than another. Last time, my estrogen level was off and I needed a different prescription. I try to exercise more instead of less; I get a massage weekly. I go to a chiropractor and make sure all my body parts are lined up correctly. I get in our hot tub. I take Advil. And sometimes I go to a lot of movies for distraction.

I don't go to support groups because I don't want to dwell on it anymore than I do. You have to find your own way. I'm available if someone wants to call me and talk about it - a group setting isn't for everyone.

Accepting that your life with chronic illness may be hard and will require planning for a time when you can no longer work:

Clela's story:

I have suffered chronic pain for what seems all of my life. Unfortunately, I look normal! I can't tell you how many times I wished my migraines and fibromyalgia would manifest themselves into some visible defect so people could see how much I hurt. I've somehow survived - in spite of failing any number of sincere attempts by physicians and alternative therapy practitioners to "cure" me by pumping my body so full of a toxic mixture of medicines and potions that it's a miracle I didn't over-dose.

Now, at age 56, I simply keep going. I've had years of practice, never having had the luxury of not working to support myself and my children. But, I have tired of running to doctors and trying one new drug therapy after another.

NOW, I try to self-educate as much as possible (using web resources for timely information); NOW I focus on keeping my strength up as much as possible with various combinations of supplements combined with only a select few prescription drugs; NOW I am trying to plan for and accept the day I can no longer work full-time and am concentrating on acquiring a state of mind that will allow me to live with the financial downturn that is almost certainly a part of my future. Though I'm not yet able to ask friends for more help and support, I have found an outlet for communicating more about my pain and fear with a fibromyalgia email Pen Pal who I have not yet met. This distant communication allows me the luxury of 'whining' without the ignoble necessity of face-to-face contact, and I find this gives me comfort.

Refusing further treatment because it is unlikely to give you a good quality of life.

Jack's story:

After a diagnosis of lymphoma, I did a lot of research on treatments I would be offered. I decided that chemotherapy was not something I would put myself through, although I did other medical procedures, including radiation. I recently learned that a cousin, who's much younger, has been diagnosed with terminal cancer. He plans to do everything to buy another year; he will have radiation and extensive chemo. I respect his decision, but it's not something I want for myself.

Leaving a support system and returning to a more conventional life.

Sandy's story:

During the first year after my transplant and rejection, I went to support group meetings every month. In fact, I even became president of one support group. After a while, though, I found that I could no longer be around people who were angry (many for very good reasons) or who seemed to have no desire to build a new and different life. So, I left the groups to begin the search for my new life.

Julie's story:

For a while, all I could talk about was my cancer. I talked about it to everybody who would listen. When I started feeling normal again and my hair started growing in again, I didn't feel the need so much. I still talk about it now, but usually just to very close friends. Recovering from the cancer treatment is still a huge part of my life. I'm not as active as I once was, I'm still on pain pills, it takes longer to get dressed and I get tired easily. But I don't want to be a cancer patient anymore. I just want to be myself. It's not who I am. I'm Julie, not a cancer patient named Julie.

Accepting death at the end of a long battle with an illness.

Gary's wife remembers:

Reassured that he had exhausted the possibilities, Gary relaxed. He was prepared to die intellectually and emotionally: sad in parting but prepared. As a professor of philosophy, for many years his classes, his community lectures and his writings had dealt with this eventuality.

With Boulder County Hospice support, he enjoyed the care and love of his family and friends at home until he died on March 11, 1998.

Some express the need to "move on" in powerful images and uncompromising advice: When Sandy was in the hospital recovering from her rejection episode, a friend sent her a book by Reynolds Price called *A Whole New Life*. Price writes about his bout with cancer of the spine and the treatment that left him a paraplegic. He admits to frequent periods of despair during the first several years as he learned to cope with paralysis and constant pain. Then, he listed some rules that helped him get on with his life. They may not be for everybody, but many people may feel this way:

> *Fairly late in the catastrophic phase of my illness, I began to understand three facts I'd known in theory since early childhood but had barely plumbed the reality of. They're things familiar to most adults who've bothered to watch the visible world and have sorted their findings with normal intelligence, but abstract knowledge tends to vanish in a crisis. And from where I've been, the three facts stand at the head of any advice I'd risk conveying to a friend confronted with grave illness or other physical and psychic trauma.*
>
> * *You're in your present calamity alone, far as this life goes. If you want a way out, then dig it yourself, if there turns out to be any trace of a way. Nobody — least of all a doctor - can rescue you now, not from the deeps of your own mind, not once they've stitched your gaping wound.*
>
> * *Generous people - true practical saints, some of them boring as root canals - are waiting to give you everything on Earth but your main want, which is simply the person you used to be.*
>
> * *But you're not that person now. Who'll you be tomorrow? And who do you propose to be from here to the grave, which may be hours or decades down the road?*

Price advises giving yourself a limited time to grieve "over whatever parts of your old self you know you'll miss." Have one hard cry, he says, then "find your way to be somebody else..." even though those around you will probably still try to find the old you. He said he wishes someone had come to him, after his five weeks of radiation and said: "Reynolds Price is dead. Who will you be now? Who can you be and how can you get there, double-time?"

Epilogue

We thank those patients and caregivers whose stories appear in this book. We are grateful for all you taught us. We thank also those who read a draft of our book and spent long hours talking to us with good suggestions.

We know that all of you are on a long journey in a life that you didn't plan on, and in a body that is less strong and less complete than you had hoped. We are on the same journey. We wish all of us courage, hope, luck, and love.

SANDY AND DIANE

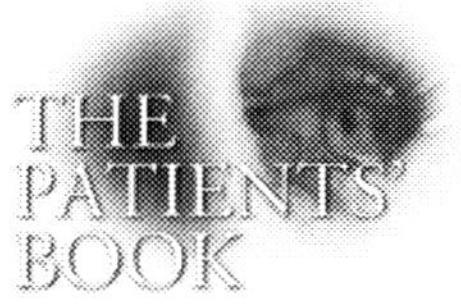

Setting the Patient Agenda

The following agendas are a collaborative effort. Sandy and Diane drew up an initial list that changed as the members of our focus groups made suggestions. Other friends who are patients and caregivers gave us their recommendations too.

1. Our Personal Agenda: What We Want from Our Doctors

- Listen to us carefully. Our stories are our part of the physician-patient partnership.
- Ask us at the outset how much information we want. For example, say to us: "if you were ever to have a serious illness seen by me as a result of a diagnostic test, how much would you want to know? What if it were a life-threatening illness, would you want to know that? What if the prognosis for your illness is poor, would you want to know that?"

- Give us a medical diagnosis or explain why a diagnosis is not possible.
- Explain our diagnosis in plain English.
- Give us copies of all of our lab tests and explain what the results mean.
- Give us treatment options and the pros and cons of the options. Tell us about treatments that do not include drugs.
- Tell us what signs/symptoms may indicate a treatment failure.
- Give us a list of the lifestyle modifications we must make to control our illness and provide us with support/motivational group information.
- Follow up on our life style modifications.
- Describe the side effects of all drugs prescribed and tell us how long it is safe to take the drugs.
- Give us the appropriate tests (creatinine clearance, body mass index) in order to determine the proper dosage of drugs.
- If a treatment option includes surgery, tell us how many similar surgeries you do annually and what percentage are successful.
- Discuss "complementary" treatments with us and be respectful of the reasons why we are interested in such therapies.

2. Our National Research Agenda

Our national agenda is the result of many conversations with patients, friends, caregivers, and medical personnel. We received many good suggestions, some of which we did not include here because we feared that a longer list might not get the attention that we hope for. Here is our own pared-down list:

- Studies to look at behavior modification techniques for the control of chronic illnesses; including the determination of what motivational strategies result in healthy life style changes.
- Studies to determine whether the use of complementary therapies in connection with western medicine increases patient compliance with physician-directed treatment.
- Studies on drug interactions. Given the sheer numbers of drugs that are prescribed for patients today; harmful, even fatal, drug interactions are inevitable.
- Standardized laboratory measurements. Patients who must switch labs because of an insurance change or a family move often find that the new lab has a whole different measurement system. Sometimes, there is no way to equate the results from the different labs.
- Studies to determine the genetic and/or environmental factors that lead to higher incidences of Lupus, Diabetes, Kidney Disease, Asthma, and High Blood Pressure in African-Americans, Hispanics, and American Indians.
- School health education programs that use the Internet to teach students how to find good health information, as well as practical ways of dealing with their own illnesses or those of their family members. (See Colorado HealthSite school programs for examples).
- Serious efforts to discipline physicians who put their patients at risk by not performing needed tests or prescribing needed treatment therapies.
- Mandatory collection and public release of data on medical errors (including a ranking of hospitals according to the number and kinds of errors), and on adverse drug reactions/interactions.

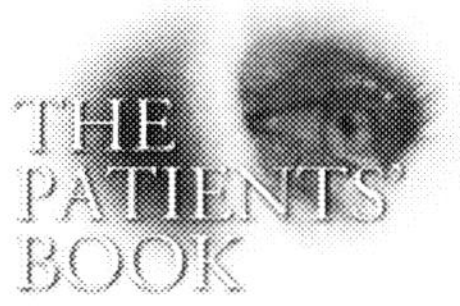

Patient and Caregiver Stories

LYNNETTE'S STORY:

(Lynnette, 33, is the hostess of the Lupus Forum on Colorado HealthSite. Please visit that forum to see her at work. Lynnette also writes book reviews for Colorado HealthSite.)

I was diagnosed with Lupus in April 1989. I had not been feeling well for months, maybe as long as a year but I attributed it to stress. I had just left a relationship of four years and I was dating again. I started feeling extremely lethargic and was losing my already small appetite. I had flu-like symptoms, severe yeast infections, migraines, blotchy skin, dizziness, ringing ears and thinning hair. The doctor I was seeing decided that I had the flu and prescribed antibiotics. He never took blood or urine tests to see if anything abnormal was going on. The symptoms would get better with the antibiotics, then would worsen again.

I tried improving my diet and exercising. It got to a point where I could not get up without getting dizzy and I was weak all of the time. I stopped eating and noticed a significant weight loss. I realized that something was seriously wrong and I was frustrated because I couldn't get anyone to believe me.

Finally, I called my mother and asked her to come and get the kids because I was too sick to care for them. I told her that my doctor insisted that it was the flu and she insisted on finding another doctor. She found a doctor that was open on Saturdays and came over the next morning to take me there.

The first thing the doctor did was take blood, urine and check my weight. While I was filling him in on my condition, the nurse returned with my tubes of blood. For some reason, I had less than half of my blood and he wanted me hospitalized immediately. Upon my arrival, I was given intravenous antibiotics and steroids and there seemed to be a sense of urgency. I was near death. They did not know what was wrong with me but suspected it was AIDS or Lupus. That was the first time I had ever heard of Lupus. Five days later I was told that it was indeed Lupus, a rare disease for which there is no cure. Lupus is a disease much like AIDS in that it's an autoimmune disease. At first, I was relieved that it wasn't AIDS but in retrospect, I don't know which is worse. In the three weeks I was hospitalized, I had two blood transfusions and was stuck and X-rayed, poked and prodded more times that I care to remember.

A year before that I had lost a baby because my water broke five months into the pregnancy and the doctors were unable to reseal it. After three days in the hospital I developed an infection and they had to induce labor. Elizabeth died about an hour and fifteen minutes later because her lungs were not developed enough. The doctors could not tell me why this happened but I suspect that I had Lupus then as well. I have not been able to carry a baby to term since.

Eventually the Prednisone they gave me bloated my body and I went from a size zero to a size 10 and began experiencing dramatic mood swings. I decided to further my education but every time I tried to pursue an education or career I developed flares that have taken months and sometimes years to overcome.

I have two forms of Lupus, discoid and systemic, and they affect my organs, joints and skin. I constantly have to reinvent myself. Where once I was reasonably attractive and productive, it has turned me into some sort of a disabled creature. The hyper pigmentation from the Lupus rashes has caused my skin to be permanently discolored and I am extremely sensitive to the sun so I can not wear anything that is going to show too much skin. My hair falls out, then grows back thinner and finer than before and is extremely fragile. My teeth are deteriorating because of bone loss from the steroids and not being able to produce enough saliva due to the medications. I have liver, heart, colon and gastrointestinal problems. I also have a circulation disorder, arthritis, carpel tunnel and chronic allergies. I usually take seven prescription medications daily for circulation, bone growth, pain and to stabilize the immune system. I also take over the counter medications for yeast infections, allergies and gastrointestinal problems.

Six years ago I had both hips replaced and a hysterectomy, all in the same year. I will soon need my hips re-cemented and my knees replaced because the use of steroids has left me with Osteoporosis and Avascular Necrosis. These operations will not take place anytime soon because I lack health insurance and/or money and have been relegated to a wheel chair for the second time in eight years. I applied for disability and was finally approved but unfortunately this does not include any type of medical insurance for 24 months. This is incredibly hard on me mentally because I am newly wed and I miss the simple things like walking down the street with my husband while holding hands or dancing. At 33 I take as much medication and operate on the same level as a 60-year-old. My doctor says that problems with my bones are my legacy and I will always have problems with my weight bearing joints.

My mother and my two sisters both have various forms of Lupus. I am afraid that my daughter will inherit this disease and had I known that I had it sooner, I would not have had children. I am fortunate to have a husband who loves me despite my physical and mental condition. While I wish I could live a normal existence, I try not to dwell on what I've lost. I am still learning what there is to gain.

POLLY'S STORY:

I've had asthma all of my life, and it has shaped me more than any other factor. Early childhood memories are of great difficulty breathing, constant visits to doctors for allergy tests and shots, missing school for up to a month at a time, almost constant fatigue, and a physically restricted life. My body reacted to any medications with terrible side effects, and frequently the doctor would come to our house to give me adrenaline shots. At that time, the doctor and my parents would discuss the "psychosomatic nature of asthma" and lead me to believe it was "all in my head." I felt guilty and inadequate and became obsessed with death at a very young age: both waiting to die and being terribly frightened when I felt I was dying.

At about age 6, lying in my bed staring at the ceiling for hours, I began to hear a tone internally. Its beauty enthralled me, and I was entertained for hours listening to it, imagining that I could ride it out of the room, the city, and universe. As a musician now, I believe that tone has been a gift that strongly influenced my interest in a contemplative type of music.

The approach to asthma treatment when I was growing up was: stay in bed and do nothing. Likewise, between attacks, I was told to severely limit my activities. As a young adult, totally apart from and contradictory to medical advice, I began experimenting with exercise (biking, walking, swimming) and the results were positive. I paced myself to work out until wheezing began, and with time, I would exercise longer and longer. I felt more energy, slept better, and felt happier. I took Yoga classes and benefited from completely changing my breathing. For the last 30 years, I have been meditating daily and believe this practice enriches my life greatly.

Since colds frequently turn to asthma for me, I spend a lot of time and energy trying to improve my immune system with vitamins, good nutrition, and often almost anything that anyone suggests. I have tried so many so-called cures on blind faith out of desperation. One of my inhalers likely has caused near osteoporosis, and I'm now on Didronel hoping to halt or reverse it.

Frequently I feel torn between wanting to escape this world and this body on the one hand, and wanting to fully engage in life on the other hand. I realize how lucky I am compared with many others with chronic illnesses. Nevertheless, I still succumb at times to depression and feeling sorry for myself.

BEN'S STORY:

I have officially been a Prostate Cancer Warrior since October of 1992 when I was 54 years old. In truth I'm certain the battle was going on inside my body for many years or even decades before that date. The first PSA blood test, done as part of a routine physical exam in late 1991, came back at 11.5 when the normal range is 0-4. Some things since then I remember all too well, some others I know must have come and gone without making any track whatsoever in my memory cells. This story is some of what I remember.

October 1992. I remember the call from my doctor saying simply that the biopsy sample came back indicating "adenocarcinoma of the prostate." The doctor's simple statement hit like a baseball bat to the stomach even though it was not a surprise. After the first biopsy six months earlier did not report any cancer, I had been living in limbo as the doctor had stated that he believed the probability for cancer was high even though he did not hit it with a biopsy needle. I've come to understand the biopsy process as being rather like searching for an unknown quantity of worms in an apple by probing with a needle.

This biopsy process had been pretty exciting, even compared to the biopsy done earlier where six needle samples were taken. This time the doctor took eighteen needle samples! Each sample is taken by driving a hollow needle into the prostate through the wall of the rectum. The driving force comes from a gigantic sounding spring — I know I shall never forget that very special "twang"!

But now we had a firm diagnosis. By this time my PSA had risen to 19.6. I did not understand it at that time but PSA over 10 is highly indicative of CaP (Cancer of the Prostate) and PSA of 20 or greater is highly indicative of systemic spread beyond the prostate. My doctor, a urologist, obviously said "let's operate," as urologists are classical surgeons and they absolutely believe in surgery. As an engineer, I wanted to know more and shifted into flat-out crisis learning and cramming. And, as an engineer my view was simply that this machine (my body) had a bad part and we just needed to find the best way to fix the broken part... as time has passed I now have a much more holistic view of illness and healing. At the time we lived in Tucson AZ which has an excellent medical school with a library open to the public. I guess I sort of moved in for a while.

What I found was too much information, too many conflicting views and opinions, and no definitive answers for a curative treatment. I did learn that CaP is tough to kill and is notorious for coming back even after the doctor says "I'm sure we got it all." And, my prognostic factors were not considered favorable for a cure. A round of second opinions showed that surgeons believe in surgery, radiation therapists believe in radiation, and oncologists believe in drugs. But it was the oncologist who was honest enough to not forecast a definitive cure as the high PSA, poorly differentiated cell structure and a high Gleason Score of 7 (an assessment of aggressive tendency) suggested to him that systemic spread had most likely already begun even though nothing was evident on bone scans or CT scans.

March 1993. I remember inspecting the cryosurgical equipment in the OR just before dropping off to sleep. My decision was to participate in a clinical trial for "cryosurgical ablation of the prostate," a procedure where the prostate is frozen and left in place, at Allegheny General Hospital in Pittsburgh. I was especially concerned that cancer was found in the apex, the lower tip of the prostate; this is an area which is very difficult to excise cleanly in a retropubic radical prostatectomy. And, there was some suspected potential that the body might produce cancer antibodies after the freezing procedure and that these antibodies may scavenge any stray cancer cells.

The protocol for the clinical trial specified that the freezing probes are inserted toward the upper end of the gland through the perineum (pelvic floor) for a first freeze and then pulled back for a second freeze in the lower end or apex where I had known cancer. When I received a copy of the surgical report I found the words "the entire prostate appears frozen with the initial freeze and the second freezing was not performed." My initial reaction was absolute despair and all I could think of was, "HE'S KILLED ME!" Maybe he did, since later examination showed the prostate had not been completely frozen, but it's also possible that the cancer was already systemic… I'll never know. I did see an attorney to consider a malpractice suit but decided not to invest the spiritual and emotional energy in an adversarial legal action. I am convinced that was, and continues to be, a good decision.

January 1994. I remember having to get up from the gurney to go to the bathroom on my way to the operating room for a Salvage Radical Prostectomy. No surprise, the cancer had come back after the cryosurgery. In the interim we had moved to Longmont Colorado and I was receiving care at the University of Colorado Medical School in Denver. It was a long, difficult surgery as there was significant scar tissue in the area from the prior freezing. The surgery successfully removed the prostate and recovery was uneventful in the doctor's eyes'; in my eyes the surgery failed terribly (as I still had cancer) and my recovery was miserable. The trip home from the hospital certainly was eventful: the transmission on the car stripped out in the middle of Interstate 25 rush hour traffic. The special help people provided to get the car to the shop and me home to my bed I will always remember.

The catheter came out in a few weeks and I no longer had to drag that special pocketbook with "the bag" everywhere I went. Incontinence continued for some months and required several biofeedback training sessions at an incontinence clinic. Like most prostectomy patients, I have reasonable control today but always wear some kind of "drip catcher" in case of sneezes and belly laughs. And, I had become permanently impotent after the cryosurgery as my nerves did not regrow as does happen in some cases. Although it's now more than five years later and I've had several hundred hours of massage and neuromuscular therapy I still have muscles and tendons which have not fully recovered from the effects of surgery. Or, maybe it's just "old age"?

March 1994. I remember: No surprise, we didn't get it all! It was now apparent that the cancer had already escaped the prostate as my PSA was 1 where it should have gone to zero when the prostate was removed. I knew then that any systemic prostate cancer is considered incurable but there are hormone blocking drugs that can delay progression. The basic idea is to hold it back long enough to die of something else first. Sometimes that strategy works. More often, in higher grade and more aggressive cancers, it doesn't. About forty thousand men die of prostate cancer each year in the United States and progress in reducing that number is terribly slow.

I have come to believe that it probably doesn't matter very much which therapy one selects for low-grade CaP as it almost always turns out OK. And, I also believe that it probably doesn't matter very much what therapy one selects for high-grade CaP as it almost never turns out OK. Maybe that's a little cynical, but with today's medical technology, I don't really think it's too very far from the truth.

Beyond March 1994: I worked my way through several hormone blocking protocols, each of which became ineffective in turn. We had bought some time but there was a price attached as well. I've lost over an inch in height, and lost a significant amount of muscle mass, gained some pounds and grown a bigger set of breasts than most girls I dated in high school. The hormone blocking drugs all shut off testosterone and that has lots of consequences. Whenever I mention the hot flashes, tender nipples and PMS feelings in mixed company I always get big grins and giggles from the gals.

By the end of 1997 it was clear that my cancer was well established in the pelvic skeleton and I had exhausted just about all the hormone blocking options. The drugs I have not yet used have greater and greater side effects and are progressively less and less effective, so for now I'll pass on those. The chemotherapy options don't look so great either... responses in some cases, usually temporary, and all the classical negative effects on the rest of the body. Some of the doctors have recommended palliative radiation as the tumor in the sacrum is pressing on nerves; this can potentially result in loss of bowel and bladder control. The trade-off is that radiation of the pelvic area generally destroys much of the body's reserve of bone marrow and of course destroys the normal bone growth and re-absorption process.

There have been countless hours devoted to investigating allopathic, complementary and alternative options which might either directly attack the cancer or just improve the body's ability to resist. One reads of so many people who have had either partial or total remission that I remain convinced that for some cases there are nontraditional therapies that work. But, every therapy which works for someone fails for others and we are quite unable to know in advance what is going to happen.

In the world of complementary and alternative therapies and things that are technically not "medicine," I have found several options to be of great value although I cannot claim a cure (the list of things which did not have value is probably longer).

Meditation and Visualization

If there has been a gift from the cancer it is in the peace I have found in meditation and prayer. In 1994 I trained in The Silva Method, a technique for meditation and visualization, which has become an integral part of my life. Some have been able to resolve their cancer or other illnesses with the power of their mind. I have not found that gift but I have certainly found a healing and resolution of the anxiety that comes with the knowledge of impending demise. I believe that is a fair trade-off. If I can recommend only one thing to others who may be seriously ill it would be to learn and practice meditation.

Body Work

Chiropractic, Neuromuscular Massage, and Reflexology have all aided in resolving physical difficulties, some associated with the cancer, some from just living. Energy Work: Reiki and Healing Touch are two methods which bring healing energy into the body and the spirit. This concept is well beyond traditional physical medicine and science but I will vouch that they make me feel better than any visit to any doctor has.

Acupuncture

For close to two years I went twice a week to an OMD (Doctor of Oriental Medicine) for treatments which generally used more than 20 needles. I have no regrets about this as I almost always felt very good after a session… I do believe that my Chi was balanced. But my cancer was not cured and in fact, I could not perceive any effect on the growth curve.

Vitamins, Herbs & Nutritional Supplements

There is great value here, but there is also great risk with this self-medication. Not everything "natural" is harmless. But, having said that, I am thoroughly convinced that we do need supplementation to obtain maximum health and resistance to illness.

Diet

From the ancient Greeks: Food is our medicine and our medicine is our food. I know that at some point in the future people will look back on this time as the dark ages of nutrition. We tend to contaminate our crops and livestock in the fields and then denature and refine our foods in factories. This is not the fuel we were designed to burn and we will continue to pay the price in reduced health and chronic degenerative diseases… yes, like my cancer!

Sharing and Caring

Very early in this journey I choose to be very public with my experience with the hope that I might be able to help others and have gone on to become an activist. I moderate an on-line mail list for alternative therapies and participate with several other on-line groups so I have contact with some three to four thousand CaP patients. I also work with the Grillo Information Center in Boulder where a volunteer staff provides one-on-one assistance in researching health issues. The Grillo Center also sponsors the Gary Stahl Lecture Series on cancer and other serious diseases. I lead an Us Too Prostate Cancer support group and often participate in a general support group at the local hospital. Even this story you are reading has been written with the hope that it might provide support for someone at just the right time. These activities do provide a sense of contribution and I know my efforts have made a helpful difference for some people.

Emotional and Spiritual Support

Last but certainly not at all the least. I thought I had the full support of my wife as a spiritual anchor while I committed myself to the battle for survival. It turns out that I was not paying enough attention to the relationship and my wife found it impossible to continue... she moved out last June and we are now in the divorce process. Maybe, if I could understand how and why this had to happen, then it wouldn't have had to happen... but I really don't think I'll ever understand. The three children do continue to provide an anchor and spiritual support for me. These few words cannot begin to express all that I feel... *what an understatement!*

Sometimes this battle feels like I'm a jet fighter pilot with a heat seeking missile on my tail. I turn and jink and drop flares but it's still there... sometimes I gain a little... sometimes it's gaining. Lately the missile's gotten really close. At some point I know it's just a matter of time and it's going to catch up eventually... but I keep on fighting... quitting is unthinkable. And now, my copilot has bailed out... a terrible sense of aloneness as I go forward to my eventual fate. But, without my copilot there is also a new sense of freedom and release to fight with even greater recklessness and abandon and even greater commitment to the battle. So it goes on, and on, and on. Maybe someday quitting will become thinkable...

At this time I think I am having partial success in limiting the spread of my cancer with a holistic cancer therapy practiced by Dr. Nicholas Gonzalez in NYC. This is a very intensive protocol which compromises three primary aspects:

1. Pancreatic enzymes which along with the immune system attack the cancer cells.
2. Detox & cleansing routines to eliminate the toxic waste from tumor breakdown.
3. Diet & supplements to restore health and balance to the body.

Dr. Gonzalez claims about 80% success for people who will follow his program. I've been on it for almost two years now and don't appear to have any soft tissue tumor although the bone mets have increased during that time. I do know others who have had better success than I have but I am continuing to work hard at keeping the faith.

In February 1999 I added a proprietary blend of Chinese herbs, called PC-Spes, to my program. In the first month it reduced my PSA tumor marker from 415 to 128 and by June it was down to 43. I was very pleased with this response but at the end of July the PC-Spes began making me violently ill and I had to stop taking it. With the sudden stop, testosterone & PSA shot up and rapid tumor growth squeezed the nerve branches in the sacrum causing some numbness and loss of bowel & bladder sensation as well as greatly increased pain level. This is pretty scary... I was picturing a wheelchair except that it was even too painful to sit.

I'm now on another hormone blocking drug, DES, which is basically estrogen. So testosterone is shut down again and breasts are filling out again. But, PSA is down to 217 and much of the numbness and pain is diminishing... life looks better again.

I have been experimenting with a number of "unproven" therapies in attempts to stimulate the immune system to seek out and destroy the cancer. Sounds like a reasonable approach but it seems prostate cancer has a remarkable ability to hide from immune attack and especially so when it's inside the bones. I continue to be optimistic that something will surface which along with all that I'm already doing will be effective... perhaps not a cure but even long term control would be OK.

Sometimes people ask how have I changed and what have I learned in my cancer journey... it's not easy to condense to simplistic statements.

- I think that people go through life being as happy or as sad as they decide they want to be. My attitude is one of the few things I have any control over… and sometimes not.
- It's hard to ask for help… but sometimes that can be a gift to those who want to help. There is support available when it's needed; sometimes you need to ask, but that's OK.
- If you wish, cancer can teach which things are most important in both your physical and spiritual life. I like the person I have become much better than the person I was before.
- Even if you have cancer you can still make a difference in the world and in other's lives. "How much time do I have?" "Enough time to make a difference," God answered.

So this is a journey which doesn't have an end just yet. I continue to work hard at the things which I think may be helping but I know some day in God's time (not mine), maybe with the cancer, maybe without, I'll go home…… and that is just the way it is supposed to be!

CLELA'S STORY:

I have suffered chronic pain for what seems all of my life. Unfortunately, I look normal! I can't tell you how many times I wished my migraines and fibromyalgia would manifest themselves into some visible defect so people could see how much I hurt. I've somehow survived - in spite of failing any number of sincere attempts by physicians and alternative therapy practitioners to "cure" me by pumping my body so full of a toxic mixture of medicines and potions that it's a miracle I didn't over-dose.

Now, at age 56, I simply keep going. I've had years of practice, never having had the luxury of not working to support myself and my children. But, I have tired of running to doctors and trying one new drug therapy after another. NOW, I try to self-educate as much as possible (using web resources for timely information); NOW I focus on keeping my strength up as much as possible with various combinations of supplements combined with only a select few prescription drugs; NOW I am trying to plan for and accept the day I can no longer work full-time and am concentrating on acquiring a state of mind that will allow me to live with the financial downturn that is almost certainly a part of my future.

Though I'm not yet able to ask friends for more help and support, I have found an outlet for communicating more about my pain and fear with a fibromyalgia pen pal who I have not yet met. This distant communication allows me the luxury of 'whining' without the ignoble necessity of face-to-face contact and I find this gives me comfort.

I do see a doctor, periodically, and have found one who is willing to listen for reasonable periods of time, readily accepts alternative therapies and who does not chastise me (much) for the many other things I should be tending to - like losing weight or exercising more. I haven't closed my mind to new options and confess that I am still sucked in (occasionally) to asking to try a new remedy. But, if nothing changes in a 60-day period of time, I give it up without self-recrimination. I work hard on trying to control my panic and think in terms of much smaller blocks of time -another day or week - not a year. I have accepted that I will remain unmarried, knowing I do not have the fortitude or patience to deal with both my discomfort and someone else in my life. I am satisfied that I WILL be able to keep going - at least for awhile!

HUGH'S STORY:
(Hugh is the host for the MS Forum on Colorado HealthSite)

I look forward to my 69th birthday in July and have had MS for at least 25 years. I was diagnosed in 1985 after I lost the sight in my left eye and began dragging my right foot, stumbling and falling when I ran, as I routinely did almost every day. I have what is now called secondary progressive MS, which means that in the early stages of the disease I had occasional exacerbations followed by remissions and then at some point a gradual, slow but steady deterioration.

I now spend much of my time in a wheelchair but can still walk short distances with forearm crutches or a walker. I have a lot of paralysis and spasticity, mostly on the right side of my body, and some pain, which I control pretty well with Tegretol. I take four medications for MS every day. I grew up in Denver, went away to school and the army and then returned to practice law, primarily litigation and trials, until I retired before planned in 1988 because of the MS. I am sure that the high stress level was a contributing cause. I have always felt a strong bond with anyone who has MS, and I enjoy comparing notes on how best to cope with the disease. I think I have learned a few things about that over the years: One is that a little humor helps and another is that self-pity does not. Beverly, my wife and best friend of 44 years, has been my lifeline to a good life in spite of the MS, and our three grown children and five grandchildren provide zest, joy and a strong sense of fulfillment. I count myself fortunate indeed.

Before MS I was quite active physically, climbing mountains, skiing, playing handball and tennis. Now I read a lot, watch TV more than I should, listen to music, surf the Internet and play chess. I'm only an average chess player, but I love it as I do Wolfgang Amadeus Mozart and Benny Goodman.

Buddies and Caregivers

MYRA'S STORY:

I believe in prayer. I believe in love. I believe every patient should have an advocate.

My beliefs are based on my experience. Two years ago my husband underwent minimally invasive mitral valve replacement surgery at the Cleveland Clinic—far from our home and traditional "support system." We knew that the surgery was risky because of his emphysema and reduced lung capacity. Without the surgery, we had been advised, he had a 50% risk of not being alive in six months. He survived the surgery (they almost always do I was told) but went into pulmonary and cardiac arrest three days later. He (we) spent 65 days in the ICU at the Cleveland Clinic, followed by 30 days in the IIC at Sarasota Memorial Hospital and three months at home with round the clock nurses. I became his advocate and immersed myself in his care—partly out of boredom, I must admit—and, because I came to believe that I could have a positive influence on his survival and recovery.

The Role of Advocacy

At the Cleveland Clinic special arrangements were made for me because I sought to be involved in his care. I was allowed in the ICU at most times—and asked to leave only when a "procedure" was necessary. I helped bathe him, change his sheets and stood by his bedside from early morning into the late hours of the evening. The nurses told me their "secrets." "I always check the monitors," Alan told me "but I also look at my patient too"!! I learned how to use the ormu bag to force oxygen into my husband's lungs, assisting the pulmonary technicians who suctioned his lungs on a regular schedule throughout the day and night. In a telephone conversation with our local cardiologist, I boasted that I had learned to "bag" my husband. He commented that knowing how to use the ormu bag might come in handy some day. In Sarasota Memorial Hospital the pulmonary technicians taught me how to suction my husband's lungs and let me practice it occasionally.

Alan's advice and the lessons learned at both the Cleveland Clinic and Sarasota Memorial Hospital stood me in good stead when I brought my husband home for the first time. We had moved the furniture out of the living room and converted it into a hospital room. My husband had a tracheostomy and couldn't speak. The home health care nurses were briefed as to the severity of his situation — he was on a pressure support machine and his lungs required suctioning regularly—and I was assured they could handle the situation. The first duty nurse seemed absorbed in her paperwork. After a short while, I looked at my husband. He appeared pale. I took his oxygen level with an oximeter and it was unacceptably low. I switched him from our oxygen concentrator to liquid oxygen, thinking that in the three months that it wasn't used, something had happened to the machine. His oxygen level went up immediately. But, when I checked him again some ten minutes later he looked in distress. His oxygen level was lower than before. I asked the nurse and her supervisor, who had arrived by then, what they intended to do about it and —while they hesitated and conferred — I said "Out of my way"—grabbed the ormu bag and forced oxygen into my husband's airways. I have been told that I saved his life because he most likely had a muceous plug in his trache which was blocking oxygen from entering his lungs. Needless to say, he returned to the hospital until we were able to field a team of IIC nurses who worked at our house on their days and nights off and were equipped to deal with the severity of his situation. Early on in this routine there was a miscommunication between me and the scheduled night nurse — she had made other plans thinking that she was off. The day nurse had been on for twelve hours already—so we decided to split the night shift between us. For six hours I was the nurse in charge—suctioning my husband's lungs, checking his sugar level and giving insulin shots as required and feeding him through the tube in his stomach—until the day nurse had rested and was able to spell me. After three months of dedicated care my husband was up and walking and eating normally, his tracheostomy and feeding tube removed.

I find that I have to carry my husband's medical records in my head. Recently, he had to have all of his upper teeth removed. They were infected and posed a threat to his new valve. Because of his medical condition, he would have the extractions done in the hospital in Sarasota. The Sarsota cardiologist wanted him to come into the hospital for a week prior to the surgery. The plan was to take him off his regular blood thinner (Coumadin) and switch him to a different blood thinner (Heparin). I knew having my husband in the hospital for a week presented the risk of infection — he is immune suppressed and had a staph infection, among other infections, while in Cleveland. I also vaguely remembered that they had put him on Heparin in Cleveland and he had a bad reaction to it. As it turned out I was right. Our local cardiologist called the Cleveland Clinic and when they checked their records they found that my husband had had a bad reaction to Heparin — (for some people Heparin separates the platelets). A call from the Cleveland Clinic cardiologist alerted the Sarasota cardiologist to a potential problem. My husband went into Sarasota Memorial Hospital the day of surgery and returned home that night. Recovery was uneventful.

The Power of Prayer

Immediately following his cardiac arrest, my husband was in a coma—perhaps drug induced. For two weeks he was unresponsive. I knew that people back home were aware of his condition and were praying for him. I prayed daily. One Saturday night I had a visit in the ICU from an ecumenical minister who had been referred to me by our Cleveland cardiologist. He was not of my faith, but I was immediately impressed by his sincerity and the force of his conviction. He said that he had come to pray for my husband. I knew in my heart that my husband could hear even though he failed to respond—and so, I was concerned that he would think that someone praying over him was giving him the "last rites." The minister, Alastair Beggs, said this would not be a problem. He proceeded to tell my husband that he was praying for him, not because he was so ill, but to speed him along his recovery. Friends who were visiting with me in the ICU joined hands with me as Alastair prayed—a simple prayer urging a steady improvement. The next morning my husband woke up and was responsive. Alastair Begg prayed for my husband twice more in Cleveland and, on a trip to Sarasota just before his tracheostomy was removed. Last November, we renewed our vows before him and friends on the occasion of my husband's 70th birthday.

Love and Family

At one point, while my husband was in the ICU in Cleveland, a young doctor, sensing that my husband was depressed and not making the effort to exercise his lungs, urged me to "Get your husband's kids up here or you could have a ventilator dependent husband."

I called his oldest son who arrived with wife and three children in tow. This visit seemed to perk up my husband's spirits and he tried harder after that. Many of the physicians in Cleveland told me that families had a tremendous impact on patients. They had seen patients that should have died pull through because family members willed them to. I witnessed one such case. After open heart surgery one patient in the ICU seemed totally unresponsive — unable to wiggle his toes or squeeze a family member's hand. He remained on a ventilator. This went on for days. But, the family never relented. They trotted in relative after relative, children and grandchildren, who held "Poppy's" hand and talked to him, urging him to wake up. After five days he did, and he made a complete recovery.

Shortly after my husband woke up, efforts were made to wean him off the ventilator. At one point, early on, a pulmonary technician took him off the ventilator, plugged his tracheostomy so that he could speak and he received oxygen only by a cannula placed in his nose. Since he had had a machine breathing for him for so long, his lung muscles were weak and the effort to breathe was excruciatingly painful.

"Let me go" he begged — meaning, that the effort was too much and that we should let him die. I held him in my arms and I told him, "I can't let you go — I just got you back." And, I have been holding on ever since.

Although my husband has no recollection of what happened in Cleveland and only a slight recollection of his stay at Sarsota Memorial Hospital, I believe that the prayers he sensed or heard and the love he felt and my advocacy on his behalf pulled him through.

GARY'S STORY (as told by his widow):

Our experience with colon cancer began in 1990 when Gary had a test where a malignant polyp was found. A segment of the colon was removed during surgery. The oncologist who visited us told us he was happy to tell us that we didn't need him: that a colonoscopy next year would be sufficient. Gary had the colonoscopy one year later, in 1991. The GI specialist reported that it was clean. He recommended that Gary repeat the colonoscopy five years later. We were so happy to have "caught" the cancer early. We believed that Gary was cancer free and that he had "escaped" the dire threat. Consequently, we looked no further. We didn't look at the statistics for recurrence or make any efforts to remain vigilant or consider prevention measures through lifestyle or diet. Gary didn't smoke. He was 15 pounds overweight but he was strong, vigorous; exercising aerobically three times a week at least, cross country skiing and bicycling from our mountain home to town and back regularly. He enjoyed a sociable cocktail and wine with dinner. We thought his diet was healthy: cereal and fruit for breakfast, mostly chicken and fish with fresh vegetables at night.

Deadly Mistakes

There was a recommendation in the written report of the 1990 surgery that we don't recall seeing: "Make a follow-up appointment with an oncologist." We believed that our primary care physicians would have told Gary to do this if necessary when they reviewed his reports. Also we kept recalling the oncologist's words in the hospital: something like: 'I'm happy to say that you don't need me.' We assumed that we would be informed and told how to watch for or prevent a recurrence especially if odds for a recurrence increased after a first malignancy. We did nothing to educate ourselves until after the trauma of a recurrence because of our enormous emotional psychological desire to believe that the threat was behind us.

Hindsight

I believe that if Gary had begun in 1990, the program that he developed after his 1994 surgery (Stage III colon cancer this time), he might have prevented the recurrence. He certainly would have been in optimum, not just good, general health. I believe that Gary's recurrence would have been discovered in time if he had been followed by an oncologist after the first surgery and if he had had annual colonoscopies.

Our Story Continued

In April 1994 Gary's primary care physician overrode the GI specialist's order to wait five years before repeating a colonoscopy. This 1994 colonoscopy clearly showed a recurrence. From the second surgery we learned that Gary's colon cancer had not only recurred but it had left the sanctity of the colon wall to float out into the lower abdominal wall and to attach to the pelvis. The surgeon reported that he'd scraped the bone as clean as possible. Treatment would require radiation and chemotherapy. I was a wreck. I am an RN and this may have been why I was so upset. I realized the implications of the extended surgery and what the surgeon was saying. My brother and a friend were with me. Thank goodness. I was nevertheless so distraught that Gary thought he would never leave the hospital alive. (I learned this later and am so sorry about this.)

We talked to the oncologist, who answered Gary's questions about prognosis, statistics, and treatment choices. I always accompanied Gary throughout his journey with cancer. A protocol of seven weeks daily radiation was followed by a "load up" of chemotherapy followed by a year of weekly chemotherapy. I called the National Cancer Institute Cancer Information Service (1-800-4-cancer). The person answering the phone was wonderful; besides phone therapy, overnight she sent us the most current information —printouts from the NCI computer database. These printouts gave the latest descriptions of all stages of colon cancer and possible treatments and prognosis. They defined terms. It remained the most useful basic information we had. Another source of good information came from a friend who searched her computer sources and turned up some solid studies of treatments and so that we could better understand the basis for the oncologists recommendations.

Gary talked to an acquaintance who was dealing with prostate and then lung cancer. His warmth and support helped Gary enormously. He took Gary with him to one of his chemotherapy sessions. He recommended books, which generally set Gary off on an inquiry into complementary therapies; making it clear that information about complementary therapies was difficult to find. After this friend died Gary pushed to start a lecture series and information center for complementary therapies. This effort was slow to start but rewarding for Gary and for anyone who took advantage of the programs. Four years later, our public library has opened a health information center for cancer and other chronic diseases that will include information about complementary therapies. Our public library, two local hospitals and the American Cancer Society support this.

Gary wanted to enter into a partnership with his oncologist. Gary wanted to do whatever he could to improve the outcome of the chemotherapies and radiation. The oncologists seemed tolerant but certainly not enthusiastic about the beneficial effects of complementary therapies beyond "don't smoke." And possibly, "limit alcohol" because chemotherapy stresses the liver and colon cancer often recurs in the liver.

So Gary consulted an orthopedic rehab physician whose holistic approach to back pain and spine irregularities had allowed Gary, for decades, to avoid all surgery and medication for a serious back problem. The physician had treated Gary's acute back pain successfully with acupuncture, exercises, and relaxation techniques. His immediate recommendation was to work with a Traditional Chinese Medicine (TCM) physician for herbs and acupuncture, change his diet to strengthen his immune system to reduce the heavy side effects of chemotherapy and radiation.

We read "Choices in Healing" by Michael Learner which gave us a comprehensive overview of complementary therapies here and around the world. Fascinating and enlightening — helpful. We decided to complement the western medical interventions with TCM herbs and acupuncture and begin systematic meditation.

We talked to our primary care physician who gave us names of several respected TCM practitioners in our area. We compared his list with the orthopedic physician's list and picked the overlapping person. Gary developed a warm and trusting relationship with this TCM practitioner that lasted the rest of his life. His advice about diet, green tea, meditation seemed extreme to us at first, but we began to notice support for his recommendations in the Johns Hopkins Medical News Letter, the Harvard Health Letter, the Tufts University Health & Nutrition Letter, the Consumer's Report on Health, as well as other journals & media sources.

Gary began daily vitamins based on Vitamins in Cancer Prevention & Treatment, by Kedar N. Prasad Ph.D. It became increasingly clear that an extremely low fat diet is important to anyone susceptible to colon cancer. When we evaluated Gary's diet, a diet that we thought was reasonably low fat, we found that this was not so. Fat slipped into his diet in many hidden ways. I took a deep breath and began to police our foods and recipes. While Gary was undergoing chemotherapy, he was unable to eat much so the first priority was nutrition, not reducing fat.

Later, I used The Cancer Recovery Eating Plan by Daniel W. Nixon, M.D. for understanding and planning our meals. After time I became adept at modifying my food prep to reduce or eliminate fat wherever possible.

Gary had used systematic visualization relaxation techniques successfully in the past. Meditation skills proved more difficult. He tried to use Larry LeShan's recommendations in How to Meditate. Eventually Gary worked with a QiGong master who enabled him to find great satisfaction in twice-daily QiGong exercises.

Gary organized a weekly discussion group with other retired members of the philosophy department. This group became the central event of his life, giving Gary a serious intellectual and professional challenge each week — unrelated to the cancer. The last meeting he attended was in our home two weeks before he died. The group continues to meet.

Not long after Gary's 1994 surgery we joined an email chat group for colon cancer survivors. This discussion group provided information about the latest medical treatments, coping with side effects, emotional support, sources for assistance with transportation and insurance. Many had sad and tough situations but real and human. Whenever something appeared in the press, we had immediate help from well-informed colon survivors who were scientists themselves. I think Gary and I began to decide against one new treatment through this discussion group because of the accounts of brutal side effects and poor outcomes.

With this information Gary and I returned to the regional cancer center's oncologist, who turned out to be the principle investigator for a clinical trial with a vaccine. From our research, we knew that this was one of the therapies we thought would be worthwhile.

Gary began the vaccine program in September 1996. Results encouraged us. The tumor did not grow. The blood marker, the CEA, lowered. No signs of spread. His liver, the most frequent site for colon cancer metastasis, remained clear.

He remained in extraordinary good health; felling trees on our mountainside; riding his bicycle. However, in mid November 1997 he began to experience some unusual back pain while hiking. A December MRI and bone scan showed metastasis to multiple bone sites. This ended the vaccine trial.

Gary and I began the search again: an updated NCI list of trials, calls to the trial coordinators. Unfortunately by mid January, Gary's general health began to suffer. He was unable to eat much at all and had GI problems. So the trials weren't an option.

During January and February, Gary continued to look for other complementary therapies: he consulted 1) a Ph.D. in ortho-molecular medicine, 2) a physician whose specialty is an aggressive nutritional program and 3) a nutrition-enzyme program. But his cancer was quickly overwhelming him. He didn't have the strength to follow through on any of their recommendations.

Reassured that he had exhausted the possibilities, Gary relaxed. He was prepared to die intellectually and emotionally: he was sad in parting but prepared. As professor of philosophy, for many years his classes, his community lectures, his writings had dealt with this eventuality. With Boulder County Hospice support, he enjoyed the care and love of his family and friends at home until he died on March 11, 1998.

References

Chapter 1

Effect of Patient involvement: Studies [by Stoeckle (1993), Quaid (1990), Todd (1989), Jones (1983), Baird-Lambert and Buchanan (1985)] [Greenfield, Kaplan, et al. 1988; Kaplan, Greenfield, and Ware, 1989]

Adverse Drug Reactions. JAMA, December 10, 1997 and April 14, 1998. In the April 14 article, the authors report that bad reactions to prescription and over-the-counter medicines kill more than 100,000 Americans a year and injure an additional 2.1 million every year.

Hospital Mistakes: LDS Hospital in Salt Lake City reported that 50% of its adverse reactions were potentially preventable, including 42 percent that happened because patients were given too much medicine for their weight and kidney function. This hospital now automatically calculates patients' kidney function daily. It has reduced adverse antibiotic reactions 75 percent and suggested that other facilities could easily do the same.

Medical Errors: To Err is Human: *Building a Safer Health System*; Institute of Medicine; advance copy, 1999.

Fosamax (Alendronate) :
Nearly one in three women using alendronate daily to treat osteoporosis complained of new upper gastrointestinal symptoms, a frequency far greater than reported in clinical trials, according to a study published in the Journal of Managed Care

Pharmacy. Of that group, 46 percent discontinued use of the drug within 10 months, more than half of them citing gastrointestinal problems such as ulcers, nausea, abdominal pain and heartburn as the reasons. The drug must be taken for an extended period to be effective.

Almost one in eight women using the drug sought medical care for gastrointestinal disorders, particularly women age 70 and older, according to a related study in the same journal. Both studies were led by researchers at Kaiser Permanente's Division of Research in Oakland, CA. The researchers surveyed and reviewed prescription data from 812 women, average age 69, who were Kaiser Permanente

"These women are typically age 70 and older," Dr. Ettinger said. "Physicians should really think twice about giving them alendronate. If elderly women are placed on the drug, they need to be monitored carefully because the risk of gastrointestinal problems is quite high."

Chapter 2

Quote from Charles Rosenberg, from Furst, *Between Doctors and Patients*, University Press of Virginia, 1998, p. 16

Quote from Dr. Jacobi, from his Inaugural Address, 1888, quoted in Furst, *Between Doctors and Patients*, p. 146

Failure of Standard Treatment Protocols, Executive summary of "Asthma in America," a national survey of public, patient, and professional knowledge, attitudes, and behavior toward asthma in the U.S. - May-July 1998.

Patients and Drugs. While patients often ask for and even demand prescription drugs, most patients do not comply with their doctor's recommendations for taking the drugs. Many studies have shown that about one-third of all patients take their drugs, one-third take them sometimes, and one third never take them. Drugs & Therapy Perspective, January 18, 1999.

Study of Incontinence in Older Women. JAMA, December 16, 1998, p. 1995

Intensive Lifestyle Changes for Prevention of Heart Disease. JAMA, December 16, 1998, p. 2001.

Prevalence of Chronic Diseases. JAMA, November 13, 1996; Vol 276, No. 18, pg. 1473.

Chapter 3

Quotes about doctors interruptions. From "How to Work With Your Doctor" by Nancy Keene and H.B. Beckman and R.M. Frankel, "The Effect of Physician Behavior on the Collection of Data," Annals of Internal Medicine, 101, no. 5 (Nov. 1984) 692-96

Chapter 5

Quote from Uwe Reinhardt - New York Times, May 16, 1999, p. 28

Chapter 6

Study on Cancer Pain. "Management of Pain in Elderly Patients with Cancer," JAMA, June 17, 1998, p. 1877. Charles S. Cleeland, PhD; "Undertreatment of Cancer Pain in Elderly Patients;" Editorial, p. 1914.

Chapter 7

Essay on Dialysis Patients, Melanie K. Landsman, "The Patient with Chronic Renal Failure: A Marginal Man," Annals of Internal Medicine, 1975.